Understanding
Diabetes

Understanding Illness and Health

Many health problems and worries are strongly influenced by our thoughts and feelings. These exciting new books, written by experts in the psychology of health, are essential reading for sufferers, their families and friends.

Each book presents objective, easily understood information and advice about what the problem is, the treatments available and, most importantly, how your state of mind can help or hinder the way you cope. You will discover how to have a positive, hopeful outlook, which will help you choose the most effective treatment for you and your particular lifestyle, with confidence.

The series is edited by JANE OGDEN, Reader in Health Psychology, Guy's, King's and St Thomas' School of Medicine, King's College London, UK.

Titles in the series

KAREN BALLARD   Understanding Menopause

SIMON DARNLEY & BARBARA MILLAR   Understanding Irritable Bowel Syndrome

LINDA PAPADOPOULOS & CARL WALKER   Understanding Skin Problems

PENNY TITMAN   Understanding Childhood Eczema

MARIE CLARK   Understanding Diabetes

MARK FORSHAW   Understanding Headaches and Migraines

Understanding Diabetes

MARIE CLARK

John Wiley & Sons, Ltd

Other Wiley Editorial Offices

John Wiley & Sons Inc., 111 River Street, Hoboken, NJ 07030, USA

Jossey-Bass, 989 Market Street, San Francisco, CA 94103-1741, USA

Wiley-VCH Verlag GmbH, Boschstr. 12, D-69469 Weinheim, Germany

John Wiley & Sons Australia Ltd, 33 Park Road, Milton, Queensland 4064, Australia

John Wiley & Sons (Asia) Pte Ltd, 2 Clementi Loop #02-01, Jin Xing Distripark, Singapore 129809

John Wiley & Sons Canada Ltd, 22 Worcester Road, Etobicoke, Ontario, Canada M9W 1L1

Wiley also publishes its books in a variety of electronic formats. Some content that appears
in print may not be available in electronic books.

Library of Congress Cataloging-in-Publication Data

Clark, Marie, 1951–
    Understanding diabetes / Marie Clark.
            p. cm. – (Understanding illness & health)
Includes index.
    ISBN 0-470-85034-5 (pbk. : alk. paper)
    1. Diabetes–Popular works.   2. Diabetes–Psychological
aspects–popular works.   I. Title.   II. Series.
    RC660.4.C535 2004
    616.4′62–dc22

                                            2003018866

British Library Cataloguing in Publication Data

A catalogue record for this book is available from the British Library

ISBN 0-470-85034-5

Cartoons by Jason Broadbent
Typeset in 9.5/13pt Photina by Laserwords Private Limited, Chennai, India
Printed and bound in Great Britain by TJ International, Padstow, Cornwall
This book is printed on acid-free paper responsibly manufactured from sustainable forestry
in which at least two trees are planted for each one used for paper production.

Contents

About the author   vii

Preface   ix

Acknowledgements   xi

1   What is diabetes?   1

2   What are the physical consequences?   11

3   What are the psychological consequences?   29

4   What about interacting with other people?   55

5   Understanding and managing treatment   67

6   Understanding and managing lifestyle change   89

7   Living with diabetes   99

8   Where can I get help?   107

Where can I get more information?   113

Index   117

About the author

DR MARIE CLARK is a chartered health psychologist who specialises in working with individuals with diabetes. She has extensive experience of working with people with chronic disorders, in particular type 2 diabetes and obesity. Dr Clark carried out a special study on developing and implementing a lifestyle self-management intervention for people with type 2 diabetes and this work formed the basis of her PhD. She works closely with Diabetes UK and is on the committee for Primary Care Diabetes UK. She currently works as a lecturer in health psychology and continues her research into incorporating both psychological research and practice into the management of diabetes to ensure optimal care and quality of life for those individuals living with diabetes.

Preface

Diabetes is one of the most common of the chronic medical disorders and is expected to present one of the twenty-first century's biggest medical challenges. The number of people with diabetes is escalating both in the UK and world wide and type 2 diabetes in particular is increasing at an alarming rate. Diabetes is also unique among the chronic illnesses in the degree to which patient behaviour influences both the application and outcomes of therapy. In diabetes, patients deliver over 95 per cent of their own care.

Diabetes and its consequences have a fundamental physical basis, but these are deeply intertwined with complex psychological issues. Such interrelationships are considerable, sometimes subtle and sometimes overwhelming. Awareness of these issues is crucial to enabling people with diabetes to lead a healthy and fulfilled life. *Understanding Diabetes* seeks to bridge the gap between the medical and psychological research on the self-care and management of diabetes in an easily accessible format and includes background information and practical guidelines on behavioural and psychological issues, emphasising personal experiences and outlining details of where further information can be found.

If you have just been diagnosed with diabetes, if you are already living with diabetes and want to find out more about it, if you are a parent, carer or friend of someone who has diabetes, or if you are interested in diabetes for some other reason, this book aims to help you. It will tell you about diabetes, its symptoms and associated problems, both physical and psychological, what causes it and how it can be treated and, importantly, how your own state of mind can help or hinder how you cope with it.

Acknowledgements

There are a great many people to thank for their encouragement, support and help in making this book possible: Dr Jane Ogden for encouraging me to write it and for her very helpful comments and feedback; Professor Sarah Hampson, who supervised my PhD, which prompted this book. I am forever indebted to all the people with diabetes who so willingly and enthusiastically took part in my research and everyone at the Chichester Diabetes Centre – in particular Lorraine Avery, Jo Wadey and Julie Grant for their boundless help and enthusiasm for my projects. Special thanks to my husband Ian, and children Anna, Oliver, Henry and Tim for their tremendous support and valuable comments and for tolerating the chaos with such warmth.

What is diabetes?

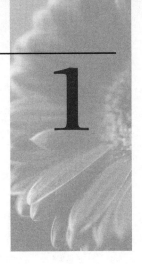

Diabetes is a permanent change in your internal chemistry, which results in your blood containing too much glucose. The cause is a deficiency of the hormone 'insulin'.

❝I just started feeling lousy, losing weight, always thirsty – it seemed like I could never get enough to drink. And there I was – diabetic! I thought my life was ruined. And then I said: 'No, dammit, this is the way I am now and I'd better learn to live with it, 'cos all of those feelings, the anger, the frustration aren't going to take it away.'❞

❝One of the most difficult things I found that I had to come to terms with when you are newly diagnosed is that diabetes is for life.❞

Diabetes is one of the oldest known human diseases. Its full name, 'diabetes mellitus', comes from the Greek words for 'siphon' and 'sugar' and describes the most obvious symptom of uncontrolled diabetes: the passing of large amounts of urine, which is sweet because it contains sugar. A proper understanding of the condition has only developed over the last hundred years or so. In 1921, two Canadian scientists, Frederick Banting and Charles Best, discovered that a mysterious substance was produced in small groups of cells, known as the *islets of Langerhans*, within the pancreas. They named this substance 'insulin' (after the Latin name for 'islet' which is *insula*), and it was probably the most important discovery in the history of diabetes. When insulin became available as a treatment for diabetes after 1922, it was seen as a medical miracle, transforming the lives of many young people who would otherwise have died after a painful 'wasting' illness.

The cause of diabetes is a deficiency of the hormone 'insulin'. A hormone is a chemical messenger that is made in one part of the body (in this case the pancreas; see Figure 1) and has an effect on more distant parts when it is released into the bloodstream. In type 1 diabetes there may be complete failure of insulin production. In type 2 diabetes, however, there is usually a combination of a partial failure of

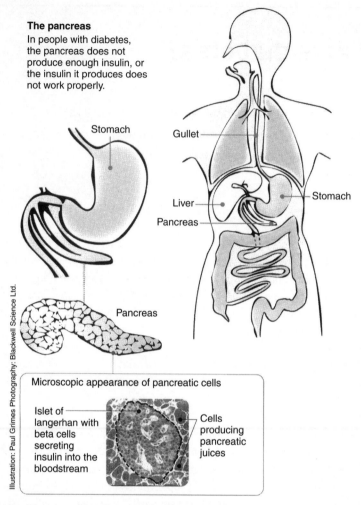

The pancreas
In people with diabetes, the pancreas does not produce enough insulin, or the insulin it produces does not work properly.

Stomach

Gullet

Liver

Pancreas

Stomach

Pancreas

Microscopic appearance of pancreatic cells

Islet of langerhan with beta cells secreting insulin into the bloodstream

Cells producing pancreatic juices

Illustration: Paul Grimes Photography: Blackwell Science Ltd.

Figure 1. The pancreas. From *Understanding Diabetes: Your Key to Better Health.* Diabetes UK Publications

insulin production and a reduced body response to the hormone. This is known as *insulin resistance*. This chapter will discuss what diabetes is and what goes wrong with normal blood sugar regulation, the different types of diabetes, what causes it, what the main symptoms are, who gets it and how it is diagnosed.

What goes wrong?

The glucose in your blood comes from the digestion of food and the chemical changes made to it by the liver. Some glucose is stored and some is used for energy.

Insulin has a unique shape that plugs into special sockets or receptors on the surface of cells throughout the body, and by plugging into these receptors, insulin not only makes cells extract glucose from the blood but also prevents them from breaking down proteins and fat. It is the only hormone that can reduce blood glucose, and it does this in several ways:

- By increasing the amount stored in the liver in the form of glycogen.
- By preventing the liver from releasing too much glucose.
- By encouraging cells elsewhere in the body to take up glucose.

Other mechanisms in the body work in conjunction with insulin to help to maintain the correct level of blood glucose. However, insulin is the only means available to the body of actually lowering blood glucose levels, and when the insulin supply fails, the whole system goes out of balance. After a meal, there is no brake on the glucose absorbed from what you have eaten, so the level of sugar in your blood continues to rise. When the concentration rises above a certain level, the glucose starts to spill out of the bloodstream into the urine. Infections such as cystitis and thrush can develop more easily when the urine is sweet as the germs responsible can grow more rapidly.

Another consequence of rising blood glucose is a tendency to pass more urine. This is because the extra glucose in the blood is filtered out by the kidneys, which try to dispose of it by excreting more salt and water. This excess urine production is known as *polyuria* and is often the earliest sign of diabetes. If nothing is done to halt this process, the person will quickly become dehydrated and thirsty. As previously mentioned, as well as regulating blood glucose, insulin acts to prevent weight loss and helps to build up body tissue – so a person whose supply has failed or is not working properly will inevitably lose some weight.

Symptoms

The severity of the symptoms and the rate at which they develop may differ, depending on the type of diabetes.

Type 1 (IDDM: Insulin-dependent diabetes mellitus)

This type starts most commonly in younger people who have to have regular injections of insulin to remain well. As the person is not producing any insulin, the symptoms can come on very rapidly as blood glucose control is lost. Insulin has a very important role in maintaining stability in the body by preventing breakdown of proteins (found in muscle) and fats. When insulin fails, the by-products of the breakdown of fat and muscle build up in the blood and lead to the production of substances called *ketones*. If nothing is done to stop this, the level will rise until eventually it causes the person to go into what's known as a *ketoacidotic coma*. This is much less common these days as diabetes is usually diagnosed long before coma develops. However, when it occurs patients need urgent hospital treatment with insulin and fluids into a vein. This is not the same thing as a coma induced by low blood sugar (or hypoglycaemia) – see page 12.

Type 2 (NIDDM: Non-insulin-dependent diabetes mellitus)

Type 2 diabetes, also sometimes known as age-related or maturity onset diabetes, is more common in middle or later life and can be controlled by tablets or just by dietary modification. As the supply of insulin is reduced or is not quite as effective as normal, the blood glucose level rises more slowly. There is less protein and fat breakdown so ketones are produced in much smaller quantities and the risk of a ketoacidotic coma is low.

Box 1. Main symptoms of diabetes.

- Increased thirst.
- Dehydration.
- Passing large amounts of urine, especially at night.
- Weight loss.
- Extreme tiredness and lethargy.
- Genital itching or regular episodes of thrush.
- Blurred vision.

Who gets it?

Around 2 per cent of people in this country have diabetes, although as many as half of them may not realise it. The vast majority have type 2 diabetes, which affects more men than women. As the age of the population as a whole is rising, type 2 diabetes is likely to become even more common during the coming years. Among schoolchildren, about 2 in 1000 have diabetes.

The prevalence of diabetes is much greater in ethnic minorities, so that, for example, more than 16 per cent of Asians in the UK may be affected.

What causes diabetes?

There are several known reasons why insulin secretion may be reduced, and any individual might be affected by one or more of them. There are many other explanations that people believe, but they are not based upon scientific evidence.

Genetic factors

Researchers studying identical twins and the family trees of patients with diabetes have found that heredity is an important factor in both kinds of diabetes. With type 1 diabetes, there is about a 50 per cent chance of the second twin developing the condition if the first one has it, and a 5 per cent chance of the child of an affected parent doing so. With type 2 diabetes, it is virtually certain that if one of a pair of identical twins develops the condition, the other will also do so.

It is difficult to predict precisely who will inherit the condition. A small number of families have a much stronger tendency to develop diabetes and scientists have identified several genes that seem to be involved. In these circumstances, it may be possible to test family members and determine their risk of developing the condition.

For the most part, however, it is difficult to identify the genes involved and this makes it different from some other conditions such as cystic fibrosis, where a single gene is operating. So even if a close member of your family has diabetes, there is no certainty that other members of the family will develop it, or if you have it, it does not follow that your children will develop it. Some people who inherit a tendency to diabetes never actually contract the condition, so there are obviously other factors at work.

Infection

It has been known for some time that the onset of type 1 diabetes in children and young people is more likely to occur at certain times of the year when lots of coughs and colds are circulating. Some viruses, such as mumps and Coxsackie, are known to have the potential to damage the pancreas, bringing on diabetes. As far as individual patients are concerned, however, it is very rare that doctors can link the onset of their diabetes with a specific bout of infection. A possible explanation for this is that the infection may have begun a process that only comes to light many years later.

Environmental factors

People who develop type 2 diabetes are often overweight and eat an unbalanced diet. It is interesting to note that people who move from a country with a low risk of diabetes to one where there is a higher risk have the same chance of developing the condition as the locals in their new country. Dramatic changes in lifestyle can also make it more likely that a person will succumb to diabetes.

A good example of this is shown by the Pacific Islanders of Nauru who became very wealthy when phosphates were discovered on their island. As a consequence, their diets changed dramatically, they put on a lot of weight, and became much more prone to developing diabetes.

All this points to important connections between diet, environment and diabetes. However, there is no precise link between developing diabetes and the individual consumption of sugar and sweets.

Secondary diabetes

There are a small number of people who develop diabetes as a result of other diseases of the pancreas. For example, pancreatitis (or inflammation of the pancreas) can bring on the condition by destroying large parts of the gland. Some people suffering from hormonal diseases, such as Cushing's syndrome (the body makes too much steroid hormone) or acromegaly (the body makes too much growth hormone), may also have diabetes as a side-effect of their main illness. It can also be a result of damage to the pancreas caused by chronic over-indulgence in alcohol.

Stress

Although many people relate the onset of their diabetes to a stressful event such as an accident or other illness, it is difficult to prove a direct link between stress and diabetes. The explanation may lie in the fact that people see their doctors because of some stressful event, and their diabetes is diagnosed opportunistically at the same time.

How is diabetes diagnosed?

❝It really scared me. My uncle had diabetes and he died when he was 40...❞

❝Finding out I had diabetes was a complete shock. There were times in the beginning when I panicked and thought I would never be able to cope ...❞

Diabetes may or may not be accompanied by obvious symptoms. In some cases, a number of symptoms become apparent very rapidly and are impossible to ignore. For example, when a person complains of going to the loo excessively, a continuous thirst and sudden weight loss, the doctor should immediately suspect diabetes. This, however, is not always the case. Some people who have diabetes do not even suspect it, because they haven't experienced any of the 'obvious' symptoms. In such cases, diabetes is discovered 'by accident' during a routine examination.

The only certain way to determine that a person has diabetes is to have the doctor measure that person's blood sugar levels. This can be done through one of several different blood tests. Some tests require that nothing should be eaten for some hours beforehand, and are usually done in the morning; some tests can be done at any time of the day, even if a meal has been taken. If the blood sugar levels are too high, it's possible that diabetes is the cause. However, the doctor may repeat a blood glucose test or take a different test to confirm a definite diagnosis.

How are blood glucose levels measured?

The amount of sugar concentrated in the blood is measured in units called milligrams of glucose per 100 millilitres of blood. The normal 'fasting' level of sugar in the blood – usually before breakfast or after another length of time when no calories are taken in by eating – ranges from 60 to 115 mg/dl in a person who does not have diabetes. After eating, the concentration of blood sugar increases, although it usually does not rise above 180 mg/dl in a healthy person. Over a period of 2 to 4 hours, blood sugar returns to the body's normal baseline. There is no such thing as a constant blood sugar level; it is normal for the concentration of glucose in the blood to vary. However, the variations that occur in people without diabetes are not as marked as the variations in people with diabetes.

What blood tests are used to diagnose diabetes?

Diagnostic tests are used to confirm a diagnosis of diabetes if there are symptoms or other indicators of the disease. For diagnostic tests, the doctor draws one or more samples of blood and sends them to a laboratory for analysis. Diagnostic tests vary according to cost, accuracy, and ease of administration.

There are a number of different types of blood tests that can be used to diagnose diabetes.

- The *fasting plasma glucose test* (FPG) is given after the patient has fasted for at least 8 hours, usually overnight. 'Fasting' means not taking in any foods or drinks that contain calories. A blood sample is taken in a laboratory or in the doctor's office to measure blood glucose levels.

- The *random plasma glucose test* – for which the patient does not have to fast – measures blood glucose levels at any given time. This is the simplest test for diabetes because it can be administered whether or not the person has had anything to eat or drink.

- The *oral glucose tolerance test* (OGTT) – which requires fasting and is administered after the patient has ingested a special glucose-containing solution – measures blood glucose levels five times over a period of 3 hours. First, an initial blood sugar is drawn to measure fasting plasma glucose levels, and the person being tested is then given 75 grams of glucose (or 100 grams for pregnant women) in a sweet-tasting solution. Blood sugar levels are measured at 30 minutes and at 1, 2, and 3 hours after the solution is given. In a person who does not have diabetes, blood sugar levels rise after drinking the glucose solution but quickly fall back to normal as insulin enables body cells to absorb glucose from the bloodstream. In a person with diabetes, on the other hand, glucose levels rise higher than normal and take a much longer time to decrease.

- In addition, the *glucose challenge test* is used to determine if a woman has diabetes in pregnancy (known as 'gestational diabetes'). It is given between the twenty-fourth and twenty-eighth weeks of pregnancy. The woman being tested is given a glucose solution to drink, and her blood glucose level is measured 1 hour later. An OGTT is usually required to make a definite diagnosis.

Summary

- Diabetes develops when an individual cannot make enough insulin or the insulin that he or she does make is either insufficient or is ineffective at controlling blood glucose levels.

- Insulin is a hormone (chemical messenger) that is critical for maintaining a healthy life.

- Symptoms of diabetes are weight loss, passing large amounts of urine, thirst and feeling run down.

- There are several causes including genetic predisposition, infections, environmental factors and stress, and any or all of these may be important in each individual case.

- Around 2 per cent of people in this country have diabetes, the vast majority of whom have type 2 diabetes.

- The prevalence of diabetes is much higher in people of Asian or African-Caribbean origin.

- The only certain way to determine if a person has diabetes is to have his or her blood sugar levels measured by a doctor.

What are the physical consequences?

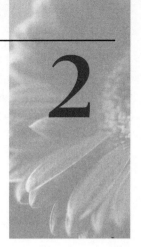

2

People with diabetes have a higher risk of developing certain health problems, or complications, and this risk is particularly high for people who are overweight, who smoke or who are not physically active.

> **"**Only when you've had it for a while and begin to develop some of the complications, then you realise that it is not such a mild thing after all and appreciate the seriousness.**"**

> **"**I now realise the different things that happen to you from being a diabetic for a long time, from the top of your head to the tip of your toes.**"**

> **"**Now I have the complications, I've had a heart attack and a bypass, only now I realise that it's not such a great thing to have after all, but you just cope and try to lead a normal life, I have to be more careful now.**"**

Complications are conditions that arise as a result of having diabetes. Some are short term, for example hypoglycaemia (low blood glucose), hyperglycaemia (high blood glucose) and ketoacidosis (very high blood glucose). Others are more long term and develop gradually over time and include heart disease, high blood pressure, damage to the kidneys, and eye and nerve damage.

However, it is important to remember that you will not inevitably develop complications simply because you have diabetes. Careful research has shown that the better your blood glucose control, the less likely you are to experience complications. Knowing this helps many people to work harder at controlling their diabetes when they're tempted to let things slide a little. Along with good diabetic control, giving up (or not starting) smoking can reduce your chances of developing complications. Smoking and diabetes definitely do not mix. All of the possible complications are more common in people who smoke, and anyone who has already developed any of the associated problems should stop smoking immediately. The importance of this cannot be overemphasised, and that knowledge may help to give you the incentive you need to stop or drastically reduce your smoking habit. This chapter will discuss the physical consequences of diabetes, in particular the short-term complications which include hypoglycaemia, hyperglycaemia and diabetic ketoacidosis (DKA) and how they can be avoided and treated. The chapter will also discuss the long-term complications, which may include heart disease, eye disorders, kidney disease, nerve disorders and foot and leg problems.

Short-term complications

What is hypoglycaemia ('hypo')?

Hypoglycaemia means low blood glucose, and in a person who does not have diabetes, the levels never fall much below 3.5 mmol/l. This is because an individual's natural control system will sense the drop, and correct the situation by stopping insulin secretion and releasing other hormones such as glucagons, which boost blood glucose. The individual will also start to feel hungry and so do the right thing by eating, which raises the person's blood glucose.

When you are taking insulin or sulphonylureas (tablets to lower your blood sugar), this feedback system no longer operates. Once you have taken insulin or stimulated its production with tablets, you cannot switch it off again, and your blood glucose will continue to drop until you have some food in the form of carbohydrate. As the level falls, it usually triggers a variety of warning symptoms (see Box 2). Hypoglycaemia is dangerous because the brain is almost entirely dependent on glucose for normal functioning. If levels drop too low, the brain starts to work less well and produces the symptoms shown in the box. If the level drops even lower, unconsciousness (coma) may result.

Box 2. Hypoglycaemia symptom checklist.

- Shakiness.
- Sweating.
- Pounding or rapid heartbeat.
- Blurry vision.
- Headache.
- Dizziness or light-headedness.
- Poor coordination.

▶

- Extreme hunger.
- Severe fatigue.
- Confusion.
- Difficulty concentrating.
- Slurred or slowed speech.
- Irritability.

How can I prevent a hypo?

Prevention is the key to dealing with hypoglycaemia. To keep your blood sugar from falling too low, eat your meals at around the same times each day – never skip meals. Recognise that hunger may be a sign that your blood sugar level is too low, and that you need to take steps to bring it back up to within a normal range. Also, make sure you take your medication as directed, in the correct dosage and at the proper times. Be vigilant about monitoring your blood sugar levels. In this way you will be able to detect low blood sugar, even if you are not experiencing any overt symptoms.

Having regular hypoglycaemic attacks is a sign that you need to go back to your doctor or nurse to see how your treatment and/or your eating patterns can be adjusted to prevent such attacks.

What causes a hypo?

You will soon recognise the situations in which you are especially vulnerable, but the most common ones are:

- Eating later than you had expected or planned, which is bound to happen sometimes. If you have had your insulin injection and then cannot eat for some reason, you should eat a small carbohydrate snack (such as a boiled sweet or a biscuit), which you ought to carry with you at all times.
- A burst of unexpected exercise, such as running for a bus.
- Drinking too much alcohol. When your liver has to break down excessive quantities of alcohol, it cannot produce glucose at the same time. This is why you will be advised not to drink too much if you are on insulin or taking sulphonylureas, and always to eat something when you have an alcoholic drink.

How can a hypo be treated?

A reaction that is relatively mild can usually be dealt with quite simply by, for example, a glass of Lucozade or lemonade. Remember, however, that diet drinks contain artificial sweetener rather than sugar, and are of no use to you in this situation. Do make sure too that, wherever you are, you always carry some sort of readily available carbohydrate in the form of a boiled sweet or a biscuit. This is especially important if you are a driver or if you are about to take some form of vigorous exercise.

What happens when a hypo is severe?

Very occasionally, you may find that your blood glucose level drops so rapidly that you do not have time to take the corrective action described above. You may become drowsy or unconscious, and might even have an epileptic fit. This is obviously a frightening prospect for you and for those close to you, and you need to take action to make sure it does not happen again. This means getting advice from your medical team to get the problem sorted out. There are various ways of dealing with a person who is having a severe hypo.

- When you are not in a state to eat or drink anything, a sugary gel called Hypostop can be squirted into your mouth or rubbed on your gums. This should not be done if the person is having a fit!
- A hormone called glucagons, which causes blood glucose to rise, is available in injectable form. You can be given an injection into your arm or buttock to revive you, and can then have something to eat or drink.

What about a night-time hypo?

It is natural for you and your family to worry that you might have a hypo while you are asleep, or even that you might have one and not wake up. This is an especially frightening prospect when you are the parent of a small child with type 1 diabetes.

In reality, the problem is by no means as dramatic as that. First, you are quite likely to be woken up by the symptoms of falling blood glucose. You may feel sweaty, restless or irritable. Occasionally, your restlessness may wake your partner even if you remain asleep. It is not unusual to sleep through a severe hypoglycaemic reaction as your body mobilises various hormones in response to the falling level of glucose, which will stimulate the release of stored glucose to correct the situation. After a reaction like this, you will awake with a headache and symptoms much like a bad hangover. Sometimes, there may be a swing too far in the opposite direction, so that your blood glucose rises too far. If you regularly wake up feeling bad with these sort of symptoms it is a good idea to take a few early morning (2–4 am) blood glucose tests to see if you are having hypoglycaemic reactions that you are not aware of at the time. At least then you will know why you are feeling so bad and you need to talk to your doctor about whether your night-time dose of insulin needs to be adjusted or altered to a different type.

What is 'hypoglycaemic awareness'?

You may well have read various stories about some people with diabetes complaining that they have lost their 'early warning system' of a hypoglycaemic reaction. Many of them believe that this has happened as a result of changing from animal to human insulin. Before we consider this aspect, we should look at other reasons why this awareness might be lost.

It has become increasingly clear for some years that people who have had diabetes for a very long time become less able to predict when they are about to have a hypo. The warning signs seem to become less noticeable after they have been on insulin for about 15 to 20 years. Although no one knows quite why this should be so, it is true that the ability of the pancreas to release glucagons in response to low blood glucose diminishes over time. Some people say their symptoms change, while others say they come on so much faster that they do not have time to take corrective action. The problem is also more common in people whose average blood glucose levels are on the low side of normal. Sometimes, adjusting the treatment so as to allow the blood glucose level to rise slightly may mean that the person gets his or her old pattern of symptoms back, but any change of this kind must be discussed carefully with the diabetes care team.

The question of what role human insulin may play in changing awareness is even more complex. While some patients feel that changing from animal insulin is responsible for their difficulties, their doctors often disagree. Carefully controlled experiments have shown no measurable difference in hypoglycaemic symptoms in people taking animal or human insulin. All the same, some people are quite sure that they feel better on animal insulin and, if so, there is absolutely no reason why they should not continue to take it.

Can hypoglycaemia be avoided by constant high blood glucose levels?

Having persistently high blood glucose levels will avoid hypoglycaemia, but unfortunately it dramatically increases the risk of developing the long-term complications of diabetes. Maintaining the balance between risky hyperglycaemia and troublesome hypoglycaemia can be very difficult for patients on insulin, but is much easier these days with the different preparations and injection devices available. If you are having troublesome hypo attacks, followed by high blood glucose levels, please consult your diabetes care team as it may mean that your treatment needs to be adjusted or changed (Box 3).

Box 3. **Key points about hypoglycaemia.**

- Hypoglycaemia can occur in any individual taking insulin or sulphonylurea tablets.
- Individuals differ in their warning signs of hypoglycaemia.
- If you think a hypo may be coming on, try to confirm with a blood test first.
- If this is not possible, take some fast-acting carbohydrate such as Lucozade or lemonade (not low calorie).
- Milk and biscuits are not ideal because they are not rapidly absorbed.
- If hypoglycaemia is a recurrent problem, seek advice from your diabetes care team.

What is hyperglycaemia?

Hyperglycaemia, or high blood sugar, is arbitrarily defined as a glucose level of >12 mmol/l. Hyperglycaemia may come on suddenly, or its onset may be more gradual, but in any case high blood sugar is not to be taken lightly. In the short-term, elevated blood sugar levels may cause diabetic ketoacidosis, generally in people with type 1 diabetes. Prolonged hyperglycaemia, lasting over the course of several years, can lead to diabetic complications such as damage to blood vessels and nerves throughout the body.

What are the causes of hyperglycaemia?

Hyperglycaemia is not always preventable, even for people who are very vigilant about keeping their blood sugar levels under control. However, it is important to be aware of the circumstances that may lead to hyperglycaemia so that you can take measures to reduce its occurrence. The causes of hyperglycaemia include:

- Eating the wrong foods.
- Eating too much food.
- Untreated diabetes.
- Lack of exercise.
- Psychological or emotional stress.

- Physical stress, such as illness or injury.
- Taking too much or too little medication.

What are the symptoms of hyperglycaemia?

Although some people do not notice any symptoms of hyperglycaemia, others experience some of the same symptoms that led to their initial diagnosis of diabetes. Usually, the warning signs of a hyperglycaemic episode include one of the following symptoms:

- Frequent urination.
- Excessive thirst.
- Frequent or excessive hunger.
- Blurred vision.
- Fatigue.
- Confused thinking.

If you develop any of the above symptoms, you should take immediate action to bring your blood sugar level under control. If you ignore these symptoms, you may have to deal with a more severe complication.

How can hyperglycaemia be treated?

The best thing you can do when your blood sugar level begins to rise is to check it more frequently. If you find that it is consistently over 140 or 150 mg/dl or if it is over 240 mg/dl on two successive checks, call your doctor and get instructions on how to handle the problem. Make sure that you are taking your medication at the right times and in the right amounts, and be very careful to follow your diet plan.

If your blood sugar is over 240 mg/dl, check for ketones in your urine. Contact the doctor immediately if ketones are present as this may indicate that you are developing diabetic ketoacidosis, a serious complication of diabetes that is discussed below. Do not exercise if your blood sugar is this high, because exercise can cause an increase in both blood glucose and ketone levels.

What is diabetic ketoacidosis (DKA)?

Diabetic ketoacidosis (DKA) typically occurs only in people with type 1 diabetes who have high, uncontrolled blood sugar levels. DKA is a condition in which the blood becomes acidic due to high levels of ketones in the bloodstream, and suggests the presence of too little insulin in the blood. If you take insulin at the proper times and in the proper doses, then the development of DKA may suggest that your body needs more insulin than you are currently taking. DKA may also develop during periods of illness or stress.

What are the symptoms of DKA?

Should you fail to recognise that your blood sugar is out of control, you may begin to experience symptoms of DKA, including:

- Loss of appetite.
- Nausea or vomiting.
- Pain and cramping in the stomach.
- A flushed appearance to the skin.
- Tiredness and weakness.
- Dehydration.
- Deep, rapid breathing.
- A fruity smell on your breath.

How can DKA be treated?

Proper medical attention is essential in cases of DKA. Do not ignore the warning signs of DKA; drink plenty of water to prevent dehydration and avoid exercise, which can cause your blood glucose and ketone levels to rise even higher. DKA often requires immediate medical attention in the hospital. The primary components of treatment are to provide additional insulin, increase levels of fluids, and make sure that electrolytes – especially potassium – do not fall too low.

Long-term complications

The possibility of developing long-term complications is one of the most frightening aspects of diabetes. Prolonged periods of high blood sugar increase the risk of complications in people with diabetes. Common ailments include cardiovascular disease (such as high blood pressure and atherosclerosis), eye disorders, kidney disease, nerve disorders, and foot and leg problems. Most of these conditions result from years of chronic high blood sugar levels. The good news is that many of the possible problems can be treated, and often the treatment is most effective when the complications are noticed at an early stage. This is why you will be asked to go for regular medical check-ups.

How does diabetes affect your eyes?

Diabetes can affect your eyes in a number of different ways.

Blurring

When you first start having insulin or tablet treatment, you may notice that your vision seems a little blurred. This is because the lenses in your eyes became dehydrated when diabetes was developing, and by rapidly lowering your blood glucose the treatment brings about a fluid shift into your eyes. This is what causes the blurring. Fortunately, the problem is only temporary and should clear up in a few months without the need for treatment. If it happens to you, wait until the blurring has disappeared before getting a prescription for new glasses, if you need one. The result of your sight test may well be different after your diabetes has stabilised.

Cataracts

When you have had diabetes for a long time, you are more susceptible to cataracts because of a build-up of sugars in the lenses of the eyes. These make the lenses of your eyes opaque, interfering with the transmission of light to the back of your eyes, and can be a particular nuisance in bright sunlight. Fortunately, this problem can be treated quite easily with a simple operation to replace your damaged lenses with plastic ones. It can often be done under a local anaesthetic, and you will normally only have to be in hospital for 24 hours. The results are generally excellent.

Retinopathy

Both types of diabetes can affect the highly specialised structure at the back of your eyes called the retina. The retina is that part of the eye that interprets visual images. It is located in the back of the eye, and contains layers of nerve cells that are sensitive to light. Diabetic retinopathy involves dilation of, and small haemorrhages in, the blood vessels of the retina. If left unchecked, these haemorrhages can scar and pull on the retina, which can cause blindness.

There are two types of retinopathy. In the milder form, known as *non-proliferative retinopathy*, high blood sugar levels damage the delicate blood vessels that nourish the retina. This may cause the blood vessels to become weak or close off, and leak blood, fluid, or fat into the fluid surrounding the retina. If the leakage affects the macula (the part of the eye where vision is sharpest), then the result is blurred vision.

Proliferative retinopathy is less common than the non-proliferative form, but is more serious. In this case, as the delicate small blood vessels in the eyes become blocked, new blood vessels form, or proliferate, in that area. In other parts of the body, the formation of new blood vessels can be beneficial, but proliferation can cause severe damage in the eyes. The new blood vessels are fragile and can rupture easily. When they rupture, blood leaks into the fluid portion of the eyes located in front of the retina. This blocks light coming into the eyes, and thus impairs vision. In addition, scar tissue can form on the retina, creating additional problems. Eye damage may become apparent shortly after diagnosis in people with type 1 diabetes, and most people with this type of diabetes (up to 97 per cent) develop some degree of retinopathy after living with the disease for 15 years or more. Retinopathy generally occurs approximately five years after diagnosis in people with type 2 diabetes. The extent to which damage occurs depends upon how well diabetes is controlled.

How is retinopathy treated?

Laser treatment developed in recent years can do a great deal to repair the damage caused by diabetic retinopathy. It is normally directed at the peripheral part of the retina, well away from the macula, and can remove hard exudates and prevent new blood vessels from growing. The earlier the treatment is given, the more successful it is, which is why it is essential that you should have your eyes checked at least once a year. An optician, a specialist ophthalmologist or a doctor who is skilled at this type of examination can do eye checks.

If you need laser treatment, you will normally be asked to attend the outpatient clinic at a special eye unit. First, drops are put into your eye to dilate the pupil to

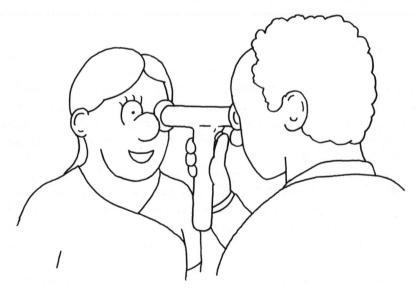

Getting your eyes tested regularly is an important part of self-care

make it easier to see the retina. You then rest your head in a special bracket to keep it still while the doctor uses a type of camera to examine your eye and identify which parts of the retina need treatment. The treatment itself is usually painless, but you will see brief flashes of bright light as the laser is used – sometimes several hundred in each treatment session. You may need several of these sessions for each eye and, afterwards, your vision could be blurred for about 24–48 hours.

How does diabetes affect your kidneys?

One-third of people with type 1 diabetes and 10–20 per cent of people with type 2 diabetes develop kidney disease after living with diabetes for 15 years or more. To understand how this complication develops, you need to know a little bit about the structure and function of the kidneys. The kidneys maintain the body's internal environment by controlling its fluid and electrolyte levels, and by removing its waste products. Each kidney contains approximately one million microscopic units called nephrons, which filter out waste products from the blood. Over long periods of time, high blood sugar levels damage the tiny blood vessels in the kidneys, making them thicker and clogged, and impairing the filtering ability of the nephrons. As a result, they are less able to filter wastes and impurities from the blood properly. Waste products in the bloodstream then build up to harmful levels. At the same time, some of the nutrients and proteins that should remain in the blood leak out of the blood vessels into the urine. The blood vessels in the kidneys can be further damaged by high blood pressure or kidney infections.

One of the substances that appear in the urine when the filters are damaged is protein and a particular protein called *albumin* appears in the urine at a very early stage of diabetic kidney damage. Albumin in the urine is also called *albuminuria* and a current test can detect the presence of very small amounts *(microalbuminuria)*. The availability of these tests is one reason why you will be asked to provide a urine sample at each of your diabetic clinic visits, even if you are normally performing blood tests for glucose. Sometimes you may get a positive result from the albumin test, which may in fact be caused by a urinary infection. Your clinic will check your urine sample to exclude this.

Your doctor will want to keep a closer eye on you if albumin is detected in your urine because there is the possibility of more serious kidney damage and even kidney failure in the long term. This is even more important if, like many people with albuminuria, you also have raised blood pressure. The two tend to go together because the kidneys also have a role in controlling blood pressure. Recent research has shown that treating high blood pressure in people with diabetes can dramatically slow down the effect of diabetes on their kidneys.

At the moment, those people who do eventually suffer from kidney failure may need treatment either by dialysis (a kidney machine) or by a transplantation, but a lot of research is being done which may one day make this unnecessary.

How does diabetes affect your nerves?

Diabetes can affect your nerves in two ways: as with the eyes and kidneys, the blood supply may be affected, or there can be direct damage to the nerves as a result of high blood glucose. Any kind of nerve damage is known medically as *neuropathy*. The consequences will depend on which of the three types of nerve is affected.

- *Motor nerves*: These carry messages to the muscles from the brain stimulating them to contract. Damage to this type of nerve is known as *motor neuropathy* and can lead to a loss of small muscle activity in the feet or hands. As a result, the toes can become clawed and stick upward and the fingers become weak.

- *Sensory nerves*: These detect pain, touch, heat and other sensations and send messages back to the brain. *Sensory neuropathy* can make the feet very sensitive and even painful at first, but eventually they will become numb and unable to feel any kind of sensation, including pain. As sensation is diminished in the toes or feet, there is the danger of additional injury and even infection. This is dangerous because you may not even realise that there is a problem, and therefore will not intervene to prevent it from worsening.

- *Autonomic nerves*: These are responsible for controlling automatic bodily functions such as bowel and bladder activity. *Autonomic neuropathy* is relatively uncommon, and its most troublesome effects are on the bladder and bowels. It can result in constipation or diarrhoea, which comes and goes, and occasionally the individual may suffer from persistent vomiting. A lowering of sexual potency may also be a problem for some men. Most of these problems can be improved by drug treatment.

How does diabetes affect sexual function?

A man's ability to have a normal erection depends upon a good supply of blood via the arteries to the penis, and on an intact nerve supply to constrict the veins leading from it. Blood enters the penis through the arteries, but cannot leave because the veins are constricted, thus producing an erection. Diabetes can affect both the blood supply and the nervous control needed to maintain an erection. It is important to remember, however, that sexual dysfunction can have psychological as well as physical causes, whether you have diabetes or not, so it is very important to discuss any sexual problems openly and frankly with your diabetes care team. There are treatments available for all forms of sexual dysfunction in men.

How does diabetes affect your skin?

Your skin is your body's first line of defence against invasion by germs and the development of infections. Unfortunately, people with diabetes are at increased risk of infection because of nerve damage, which makes repeated injury to the skin more likely. Poor circulation also contributes to the risk of infection, since blood and nutrients cannot reach the site of injury to help in the healing process.

A small minority of people with diabetes may have skin problems caused by damage to the small blood vessels. When this occurs, it results in reddening and thinning of the skin over the lower shinbones – a condition known as *necrobiosis lipoidica*. Unfortunately, there is no effective treatment. Other skin-related problems that are statistically more likely to occur in people with diabetes include fungal infections, a depigmentation of the skin called *vitiligo*, and loss of hair on the head, known scientifically as *alopecia*.

How does diabetes affect your feet?

You need to be aware of changes to your feet that can arise because of your diabetes and of what you can do to minimise the risk of damage. Most people with diabetes do not get serious foot problems, but even those who do can prevent the problem worsening by caring for their feet properly. Healthy circulation to your feet will help to keep the tissues strong, and you can encourage this by eating the right kinds of foods, keeping good control of your diabetes and by not smoking. Ensure that your shoes fit well with enough room for your toes, and with a fastening to keep them in place without rubbing. In addition, there are specific things you can do to look after your feet. These are designed to guard against four changes, which can be caused by diabetes.

- *Poor blood supply*: The result of the blood vessels becoming narrower. When your circulation is restricted in this way, your foot is less able to cope with hazards like cold weather, infection or injury, and is more susceptible to the other three changes below. Keep your feet warm with good-quality socks and stockings but avoid overheating; and be very careful of seams in your socks that can press and rub, causing blisters. Consider wearing the socks inside out if the seams are prominent.

- *Neuropathy*: Neuropathy makes the foot less sensitive to pain and temperature. In its early stages, people often complain of pins and needles or a feeling that they are 'walking on cotton wool or pebbles'. When the ability of your foot to feel is reduced, you are less likely to notice accidental injuries or infection which will lead to increased damage if no remedy is applied. In some cases, skin breaks down over the part of the foot that has experienced sustained pressure, because you do not feel the discomfort that would otherwise make you shift your position. If you are suffering from some degree of neuropathy, you need to get into the habit of checking your feet every day for any cuts or wounds that did not hurt you at the time. The easiest way is to make a regular foot care programme part of your daily routine. It is also important to check the water temperature with your hand before getting into a bath, and to avoid 'toasting your toes' in front of the fire.

- *Dryness*: Loss of elasticity or dryness in the skin of your feet can be associated with neuropathy and a poor blood supply, but it can develop even when you have good circulation and a normal amount of feeling. You may notice your skin becoming dry even if you have not had diabetes for very long, and be inclined to dismiss it as just a minor nuisance. However, dry and flaky skin is much less supple because sweat and natural oils from the everyday pressures and frictions of walking do not protect it. When the skin on your feet is very dry, you are more prone to the formation of calluses and corns, and also to splits around the edges (known as fissures). You can help to replace some of the lost natural moisture by applying a good hand cream every day and using a foot file or pumice to remove dead skin. However, be gentle, and never use chemicals designed to remove corns and calluses or try to cut them away with blades because you could easily injure yourself.

- *Changes in the shape of your feet*: These can take place over a period of time as a result of diabetes. The bones underneath may become more prominent due to changes in the fatty pad under the ball of your foot. The front part of your foot may spread and your toes may claw. When the tissues under your foot are strained, you may get pain in your heel. Usually these changes are a result of minor alterations in the shape of your foot, but do not forget that they could still indicate that you need new shoes for a better fit.

Expert care

As a person with diabetes, you are eligible for treatment from a state-registered chiropodist (also called a podiatrist) on the NHS – your GP, health centre or diabetes centre should have a list of local practitioners. Many people are perfectly able to look after their own feet, but anyone who has a physical or visual disability, or any of the complications listed above, should have regular appointments with a state-registered chiropodist.

How does diabetes affect your heart?

People with diabetes are two to four times more likely to develop cardiovascular disease than people who do not have diabetes, and are five times more likely to have a stroke. Statistics show that more than half the deaths in older people with diabetes are due to cardiovascular disease. Most of the complications occur when blood vessels become too narrow or are clogged, or the blood itself becomes too thick. This reduces or even blocks blood flow to the heart, brain and other important parts of the body. When blood flow to the heart is slowed for a period of time, one result is a kind of chest pain called *angina*, and this is a warning signal that something is reducing the flow of blood to the heart. Two types of cardiovascular complications that can result from diabetes are hypertension (high blood pressure) and atherosclerosis (hardening of the arteries).

Blood pressure

Blood pressure, the force exerted by the blood against arterial walls, is what keeps blood circulating. If the pressure is too high, it places a strain on the arteries that can lead to serious problems throughout the body. Of all the risk factors for cardio-vascular disease, high blood pressure is one of the greatest. High blood pressure is very common among people with diabetes. In many cases, the condition does not produce outward symptoms, so many people are not even aware that they have it. Therefore, high blood pressure may go undiscovered until detected during a routine physical examination or an examination for another heart problem. It is estimated that 60 per cent of people with type 2 diabetes may have high blood pressure.

High blood pressure damages coronary arteries and forces the heart to work harder than it should. It also contributes to *atherosclerosis*, or hardening of the arteries, and increases the risk of heart attack. This is why it is so important for anyone who has high blood pressure, especially if he or she has diabetes, to bring the condition under control since it can contribute to other diabetes complications such as kidney or nerve damage.

Atherosclerosis

Atherosclerosis occurs when plaque, which is made up of fat and cholesterol, becomes deposited on the walls of the arteries and, to a lesser extent, the veins. This narrows the blood vessels, and eventually makes them hard and inelastic. If measures are not taken to reverse plaque build-up, the blood vessels can become so narrow that they clog easily, preventing the blood from carrying oxygen and nutrients to body tissues.

People with diabetes have an increased risk of developing atherosclerosis, because of the interaction of a number of factors but most importantly because high blood glucose affects the tissue that lines the inner surfaces of the coronary arteries. This causes the release of harmful chemicals that create a sticky surface and makes the inner walls of the arteries more susceptible to plaque formation. When atherosclerosis develops, it affects not only the coronary arteries but also all the other arteries. When the arteries in the brain become seriously narrowed, the result is a stroke. The vast majority of strokes occur because of arterial blockage. In the legs, serious atherosclerosis is known as *peripheral vascular disease*. Peripheral vascular disease is an underlying factor in the development of many of the lower leg and foot problems associated with diabetes. As the plaque builds up, blood flow to the lower legs and feet is decreased.

HELPFUL TIPS! HELPFUL TIPS! HELPFUL TIPS! HELPFUL

There are various ways of 'handling' risks of heart disease:

- You can reduce your risk of heart disease by controlling your blood glucose, cholesterol and other blood fats, keeping your blood pressure within a healthy range, and managing your weight.

- Your diabetes treatment programme should include a healthy eating plan and a programme of regular physical activity, which will help you to achieve these goals.

- By including low-fat, high-fibre foods in your diet, you can significantly lower the level of fat in your blood.

- Research has also shown that fibre binds with certain substances that would normally result in the production of cholesterol, and eliminates these substances from the body. In this way, a high-fibre diet helps to lower blood cholesterol levels, reducing the risk of heart disease.

- It is also important to avoid habits that increase the risk of heart disease, such as smoking.

Finally

You are probably feeling rather alarmed after reading about all these possible complications, so it is worth emphasising again that they can all be prevented by careful attention to diabetes care and blood glucose control. Remember that complications are not inevitable, and that you have an important role to play in preventing the occurrence of complications.

Summary

- People with diabetes have a high risk of developing complications, some of which are short term: for example, hypoglycaemia (low blood sugar levels), hyperglycaemia (high blood sugar levels) and ketoacidosis (very high blood sugar levels).

- Other complications are more long term and develop gradually over time and include heart disease, high blood pressure, damage to kidneys, eyes and nerves.

- Two types of heart disease complications that can result from diabetes are atherosclerosis (hardening of the arteries) and hypertension (high blood pressure).

- Kidney damage occurs in a minority of people and can be detected early by a urine test for albumin.

- Diabetes can affect the eyes by causing cataracts or damage to the back of the eyes called retinopathy; early detection and treatment are very effective at preventing progression and loss of eyesight.

- Nerves can also be damaged and feet and hands need to be checked regularly. Foot care is extremely important in preventing complications and feet should be checked at least once a year by a health-care professional.

What are the psychological consequences?

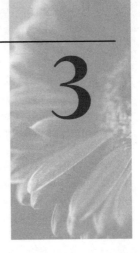

3

As well as the physical consequences, the diagnosis of diabetes can have a tremendous psychological impact on you, affecting your family, your friends and almost everyone around you.

> 66When I was first diagnosed it was very dramatic, it was really frightening, the fear of the unknown really. 99

> 66I don't think it's all that devastating, there are far worse incurable sorts of things. 99

> 66It was easy for me because my son had it, so I had the experience of it, I knew what it was already. 99

Each person's responses to a diagnosis of diabetes are different. Even your own reactions to the condition will vary from time to time. This chapter will discuss, first, how people attempt to make sense of the diagnosis and try to understand the implications of having diabetes, and then consider some of the common emotional reactions to diagnosis including denial, anxiety, relief, depression, anger and stress, providing some helpful tips for coping with these common emotional reactions.

How do you feel about having diabetes?

Your emotions can be like a roller coaster, and ups and downs are very common. Your emotional reactions to diabetes may start even before treatment begins. Of course, how you react will depend partly on how suddenly your condition develops, but there are many other factors that influence your reactions to diagnosis and living with diabetes, which makes it very difficult to predict just how a person will react at any given time. How did you handle problems before your diabetes was diagnosed? What was your general coping style? Were you calm or nervous? Were you persistent or did you give up easily? The way you have handled life's problems in general will suggest how well you will cope with diabetes and its treatment. Your age will also have a bearing on how you respond emotionally. Your general physical health prior to the onset of diabetes will also play a role in determining your coping ability, as will your relationships with your family and friends.

Immediately after diagnosis, people are often in a state of shock. They find that their usual ways of coping with problems do not work, at least temporarily, and they may experience intense feelings of disorganisation, anxiety, fear and other emotions. Eventually this crisis phase passes and people begin to develop a sense of how the diabetes will alter their lives and can be integrated into them. At this point, more long-term difficulties that require ongoing attention may become apparent.

Making sense of the diagnosis

Personal models of illness are people's beliefs and emotions about their disease. In the same way that people have beliefs about health, they also have beliefs about illness. Psychologists have shown that these beliefs appear to follow a pattern and are made up of (1) beliefs about the diagnosis and symptoms, (2) beliefs about the seriousness of the condition, (3) beliefs about how long it will last, (4) beliefs about what caused the condition, and (5) beliefs about whether it can be cured or whether the condition requires medical intervention.

Of the many beliefs that people hold about their illness, two in particular are thought to relate to long-term adjustment: beliefs about the cause of their illness ('Why did it happen?') and beliefs about whether or not the illness can be controlled ('What can I do to manage it now?').

Why did it happen?

A large number of researchers have noted that people suffering from both acute and chronic illness develop theories about how they contracted their illnesses. Individuals' theories about the origins of chronic illnesses, like diabetes, include stress, physical injury, disease-causing bacteria, and God's will. Importantly, where people place the blame for their illness is highly significant. Do they blame themselves, another person, the environment, or a quirk of fate?

Self-blame

❝I suppose if I paid more attention to my weight and that, it might not have happened, so I do blame myself a bit for it happening.**❞**

> ❝Well, it's down to me, isn't it, I mean I've always smoked and I never do any exercise really, so I suppose if I had looked after myself a bit better like they tell you to, yes, I do blame myself for this [*diabetes*].❞

Self-blame for chronic illness is widespread. People frequently perceive themselves as having brought on their diabetes by their own actions. In some cases, these perceptions are to a certain extent correct. Poor health habits such as smoking, improper diet or lack of exercise can cause illnesses like heart disease, for example. But what are the consequences of self-blame? Unfortunately, there is no straightforward answer to this question. Some researchers suggest that self-blame can lead to guilt, self-recrimination or depression. Self-blaming individuals may be poorly adjusted to their illness because they focus on things they could have or should have done to prevent it. On the other hand, other research suggests that self-blame may be adaptive. Perceiving the cause as self-generated may represent an effort to assume control over the disorder; such feelings can be adaptive in coping with and coming to terms with the disorder. It may be that self-blame may be adaptive under certain conditions and not under others.

Understanding the cause of the illness and developing an insight into the implications of the illness gives the illness meaning. A sense of meaning contributes to the process of coping and adapting to your diabetes.

What can I do to manage it now?

> ❝... and it sure would have helped if someone had told me **I** was in control, even though my diabetes was out of control. I never saw that **I** was the one who went on binges or 'forgot' my medication. It just sort of happened, like someone else was doing it to me.❞

> ❝I really believed that insulin was the answer, that if only I could get on to insulin then I wouldn't have to think about it, I could sort of hand it over, and the insulin would be in control.❞

Researchers have also examined whether people who believe they can control their diabetes are better off than those who do not see their diabetes as under their control and people develop a number of control-related beliefs with respect to their condition. A sense of control can be achieved either through psychological techniques such as developing a positive attitude, meditation, self-hypnosis or a type of causal attribution, or by behavioural techniques such as changing diet, changing medications, accessing information or controlling any side-effects. These processes contribute to a sense of 'mastery' over the diabetes.

Coping strategies

In many ways, coping with a diagnosis of diabetes is like coping with any other severely stressful event. Research suggests that appraisal of a chronic disease as threatening or challenging leads to the initiation of coping efforts. Which strategies facilitate best psychological adjustment? There is some evidence that, like coping with other stressful events, the use of avoidant coping is associated with increased psychological distress, and thereby may be a risk factor for adverse responses to illness. Similarly, poor adjustment has been associated with efforts to forget the disease, fatalism, passive acceptance, withdrawal from others, blaming of others and self-blame, and this form of coping has also been related to poor blood glucose control. In contrast to this, research has found lower psychological distress to be associated with positive, confrontative responses to stress and with beliefs that one can personally direct control over an illness.

Emotions

> ❝I did think, is this what I have to look forward to, is this all there is to life. I know insulin makes it easier these days but it's like a life sentence, and I worry that I will get like my mother.❞

It is very common to feel overwhelmed after learning that you have a condition such as diabetes; there is no easy way to accept the fact that your life is going to change. When first diagnosed, you may not be able to react at all, since it may not seem 'real' to you, especially if you don't have any noticeable symptoms. As the full impact of the diagnosis sets in, you may experience a whole variety of feelings ranging from sadness and anxiety to anger and frustration. You may feel upset because you will need to make some lifestyle changes, and you may be afraid that you will never adjust to living with diabetes.

Denial

> ❝I just don't want to know about this diabetes. I wish it would just go away, ever since they told me I had it. As far as I am concerned I just ignore it, pretend it isn't there, then maybe it will go away.❞

> **"**I don't take it very seriously, sort of deny it's there really, I just deal with all the other events in my life and dismiss diabetes, I'm not working with it.**"**

It is not at all unusual to deny that a problem exists. Regardless of the symptoms you have been experiencing, hearing that you have diabetes may provoke denial. Denial is especially risky in the case of diabetes. People who deny that the problem exists will not take steps to treat the condition and poorly controlled diabetes can lead to any number of short- and long-term complications.

There are two main ways that people with diabetes may act out their denial. First, there is denial that part or all of the treatment programme is necessary. If this is the case, you might completely disregard all of the components of your diabetes management plan. Some people ignore certain aspects of treatment, but adhere to others – for example, taking medication but not eating properly. Second, there is denial that symptoms may suggest a progression of the illness or the development of a diabetes-related complication. For instance, a person who is experiencing blurred vision may not report this symptom to his or her health care team. This may be an attempt to delay the doctor's discovery of a more serious problem.

However, denial can also serve as a protective function. It has been shown, for example that denial can protect an individual, immediately after the diagnosis of illness, from having to come to terms with the full range of problems posed by the illness at a time when he or she may be least able to cope with it. Denial can also reduce the experience of the unpleasant symptoms and side-effects of treatment, and mask the fear and worry associated with a chronic disease, until you are more accustomed to the diagnosis and better able to sort out realistically the restrictions it will impose.

Overall, then, denial may be useful in helping people to control their emotional reactions to illness, but importantly it may interfere with their ability to monitor their conditions, to take the initiative in seeking treatment, or to follow through when they must act as responsible co-managers of their illness.

Anxiety

> **"**I feel so afraid, no peace or in control.**"**

> **"**I keep thinking that something bad is going to happen, something I have to protect myself from. I feel so vulnerable the whole time.**"**

Immediately after the diagnosis, a commonly experienced reaction is anxiety. Anxiety is a problem not only because it is intrinsically distressing, but also because it can interfere with good functioning. Anxious patients may be debilitated by their emotional distress even before treatment begins – for example, anxious diabetic people report poor glucose control and increased symptoms.

Anxiety is high when people are waiting for test results, receiving diagnoses or waiting for medical procedures and anticipating the adverse side-effects of treatment. Anxiety is also high when people expect substantial lifestyle changes to result from an illness or its treatment, when they feel dependent on health professionals, and when they lack information about the nature of the illness and its treatment.

While anxiety that is directly attributable to the illness may decrease over time, anxiety about possible complications, the disease's implications for the future and its impact on work and social activities may actually increase.

Relief

"I remember noticing with surprise that I felt a strong sense of relief, at last I knew why I'd been feeling so listless and unwell for all those months. It was a comfort to know what was wrong and that someone understood what was happening to me.**"**

"I was relieved with the diagnosis, that there was a name put to the disease and they can do something about it.**"**

Some people are actually relieved when they are diagnosed with diabetes, usually because they know there is a problem but do not know what it is. If some people are experiencing different symptoms and nothing seems to help, then the diagnosis of diabetes may give them hope that treatment will improve the way they are feeling. Perhaps they think that their symptoms are 'purely psychological', in which case it is better to learn that there is a reason for why they have been feeling poorly and that it is not all 'in the head'.

Depression

"I feel so down and hopeless. I certainly didn't ask for diabetes and now so many changes have to be made in my life. I worry about the future and whether I'll get any of the complications, I'm just so helpless.**"**

"What good am I? I'm not helping anybody around me, and I'm not helping myself. I just feel really useless.**"**

❝I do worry about the future because I have relatives with diabetes and see what's happened to them. I don't want to end up like that, it's a bit depressing really.**❞**

Depression is a serious problem. It is three times more common in individuals with diabetes than in the general population, affecting at least 15 per cent of people with diabetes. Depression is a concern not only because of its mental health implications, but also because of its negative impact on self-management, glucose control and complications in both adults and children. Yet, in people with diabetes, depression is often underdiagnosed.

What are the symptoms of depression?

There are a number of possible symptoms of depression. If you notice that you are feeling excessive amounts of sadness, discouragement or melancholy, or if you are unable to eat and this problem has nothing to do with the diabetes or its treatment, or if you are sleeping either too much or too little, or if you feel totally withdrawn from social activities, or if you find yourself crying often and it is not your typical behaviour, or if you are brooding about the past and feeling hopeless, then any of these feelings may indicate depression.

There are many other symptoms. If you are experiencing excessive amounts of irritability or anger, or if your fears seem to be extreme, or if you feel inadequate and worthless, or if you are unable to concentrate on virtually anything in your life, whether it be work, family or other interests, or if you seem to have little or no interest in activities that previously gave you pleasure, or if you have reduced amounts of energy that do not seem to be related to the disease or treatment, or if you have little or no interest in sex or intimacy, or if the way you think, speak and act seems to be generally slowing down, then any of these can also be symptomatic of depression. The more of these symptoms you experience, the more likely it is that you are depressed and should take some action to help yourself.

How can you cope with depression?

Importantly, remember that high blood sugar can make your depression worse; therefore, one of your first steps towards alleviating the depression should be to bring your blood sugar under tight control, if you have not already done so.

The strategies and techniques that are most effective in dealing with depression can also be effective in preventing you from becoming depressed. Unfortunately, this does not mean that you will never again feel depressed. It may not happen, but if it does recur you will know that you can do something about it.

There are various ways of 'handling' depression: for example, being more physical (in other words, doing something), working on your thinking, and discussing it with others.

- **Getting physical**. There are two ways of getting physical in order to deal with depression: actively working to accomplish goals, and increasing physical activity. Unknowingly, you may be using a lot of energy to keep yourself depressed. You may be working hard to keep that anger inside, even if it appears to others that you are simply withdrawing. If your depression is anger turned inward, then by releasing your anger you may be able to eliminate your feelings of depression. However, you must find an object towards which your anger can be expressed, and this may be difficult.

- *What kinds of activities can help you to release your anger?* Many physical activities can be effective. Exercise helps by lowering your blood sugar level, and it also causes the release of neurotransmitters called *endorphins*, which make you feel good and give you a more positive attitude. Remember, before you begin any exercise programme, it is very important that you work closely with your diabetes care team to plan a programme that is safe for you and will provide maximum benefits with little or no risk.

- **Thinking traps**. Although getting physical may help to lift your depression, and can also provide a great distraction, which may help you to look more objectively at what is going on, physical activity alone will not teach you ways of fighting inappropriate thinking. Remember that it is your *thoughts* that have made you depressed. Clearly, restructuring your thinking is a key element in alleviating depression and dealing with any negative emotion.

- *When you are depressed, psychological research suggests that you tend to distort reality.* It is important to recognise, therefore, that your thoughts are not necessarily based on what is really happening, but may instead be based on your own distorted views. This is called *cognitive distortion*: 'cognitive' refers to your thinking, 'distortion' means that you are twisting things around and in general losing sight of what is real. We all tend to do this from time to time, but when you are depressed, you do it most of the time, and this is what keeps you depressed.

- *Make sure you know what is true and what is not.* Provide your own assessment of the situation, and be as objective as possible. Then, if necessary, ask other people – those whose opinions you trust – for their evaluation. Right now, you may be better off accepting somebody else's perceptions of the situation, because that person is probably more objective and more accurate. Work to become more comfortable with any differences in perception and to adjust your thinking so that it more closely resembles the actual circumstances. Since so many feelings of worthlessness are based on distorted facts, depression can be reduced, if not eliminated, once these facts are straightened out.

- *Remember, everyone has problems but if you are depressed, you may feel overwhelmed.* Once you begin to feel depressed, your negative thoughts will soon lead to negative actions. These negative actions will lead to more negative thoughts, which will in turn lead to more negative actions, and so on. It is an ongoing, vicious cycle that will spiral you further downward into deeper depression. Eventually, you will feel trapped in this vicious cycle, and may believe that there is no way out. Do your best to view each problem objectively, and avoid blowing it out of proportion. Try to think positive thoughts. If you find yourself unhappily comparing your present life to life before diabetes, try to modify your thinking. Start planning fun things for the present and future. But this takes effort; do not wallow in self-pity, because that will only allow your depression to overwhelm you. Develop some positive plans, and translate them into pleasure! Remember: your thoughts lead to your emotions. If your thoughts are negative and critical, your emotions will be the same. But if you can turn your thoughts around to a more positive, constructive point of view, your emotional reactions will almost certainly follow.

- **Talk about it**. Most importantly, you should talk about your problems and concerns with others and definitely consider speaking to your diabetes team. You may be referred for counselling, which is a very effective way to treat depression, but in a small percentage of cases, depression may be caused by biochemical deficiencies or chemical imbalances in our bodies. So, if your depression is persistent and non-medical coping strategies are not effective, then antidepressant medications may be recommended.

- *Modify your thinking.* Regardless of whether your depression is caused by a biochemical deficiency or by your reaction to the people and events around you, you should still try to modify your thinking. Many experts believe that even if the cause of depression is biochemical, by working on the way you handle your day-to-day living you can have a positive effect on your emotions.

Anger

❝I am fed up with the whole thing. I am sick and tired of watching what I eat, or people telling me I should be. I am fed up with having to check my blood sugar every day and sick of giving myself injections. The whole thing just makes me so angry.❞

❝My feelings were very mixed. I felt stunned and angry, cheated out of my health, and I couldn't believe that the diagnosis was correct.❞

In general, people with any chronic medical problem may be angry. These feelings are often exacerbated if the illness requires extra self-care. Because anger results in the build-up of physical energy that needs to be released, in other words stress, it is important to learn how to cope with this emotion.

Just what is anger?

When you have a desire or goal in mind and something interferes with your efforts to reach it, this can be very frustrating. A feeling of tension and hostility may result, which is what we refer to as anger. In learning to cope with your anger, you must realise that anger exists uniquely in the mind of each angry individual. Anger is a direct result of your thoughts, not of events. An event in and of itself does not make you angry. Rather, your anger is caused by your interpretation of the event, the way you think or feel about it.

Are there different types of anger?

In learning to deal with anger, it can be helpful to discuss the three different ways in which anger can be experienced. This may enable you to more easily identify anger when it does occur.

The first type of anger is *rage*, the expression of violent, uncontrolled anger. This is probably the most intense anger you can experience. It is an outward expression that results in a visible explosion. Often, rage can be a destructive release of the intense physical energy that has built up over time.

The second type of anger is *resentment*. This feeling of anger is usually kept inside, a growing, smouldering feeling of anger directed towards a person or object but is often kept bottled up. Resentment tends to sit uncomfortably within you and can do even more physiological and psychological damage than rage.

The third type of anger is *indignation*, and this is often regarded as a more appropriate, positive type of anger. Unlike rage, it is released in a controlled way.

Obviously, these three types of anger can occur in combination and in many different ways. Understanding the different ways of experiencing anger can help you to identify and cope with it when it does occur.

What causes anger?

For some people with diabetes, the extra self-care that diabetes management requires can certainly be a source of anger. You may be angry because you feel that you cannot eat what you want. You may become angry if you believe that your diabetes has imposed limitations on your life. You may get angry if you feel that your family is not understanding enough, or you may think they are trying too hard to protect you. Or you can become frustrated if you cannot seem to keep your blood sugar under control no matter how hard you try, and this may cause you to feel angry. Thoughtless comments from others can also cause anger. You must, of course, become aware of anger before you can deal with it and realise that resolving your anger will not make your diabetes go away.

Why me?

One of the common questions that people with diabetes ask is 'Why me?' This question suggests that what has happened should not have happened, that it is unfair, or that someone or something is to blame. It is important to realise that, in this case, anger is not helpful; that asking 'Why me?' will not benefit you in any way. It is far better to ask yourself what you can do about it now that it has happened.

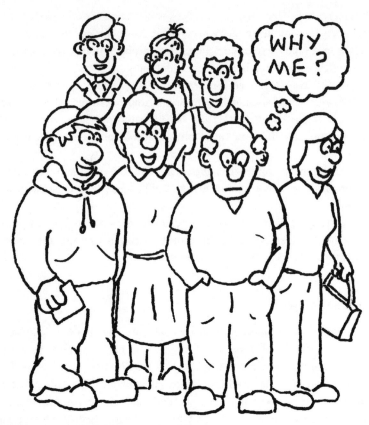

Coming to terms with diabetes can be difficult

HELPFUL TIPS! HELPFUL TIPS! HELPFUL TIPS! HELPFUL

There are various ways of 'handling' your anger:

- If you feel overwhelmed by the intensity of your anger, and fear that you may completely lose control, you may try to do whatever you can to avoid the experience. This might include pushing any angry thoughts out of your mind, no matter how important the issue. In the long run, however, this would not be regarded as the best way to deal with anger.

- It is possible to see anger as a necessary, though unpleasant, part of life. You know that there will be times when you will be angry, whether you like it or not. But you can choose to deal with both your anger and the situation that is causing it as effectively as possible. Your own reaction to anger is unique. It may also change from time to time. There may be times when you accept anger and almost value it as a motivator. At other times you may attempt to push it away. Of course, the way in which you deal with your emotions now that you have diabetes is probably similar to the way in which you have dealt with them in the past. If you have always dealt with problems in a generally positive, constructive manner, you will probably deal with new problems in the same way. On the other hand, if you have had difficulty dealing with stress in the past, you may also have problems dealing with it now.

- As you learn to cope with your anger, it is important to remember that events alone do not make you angry. It is your thinking, your interpretation of these events, that leads to anger. And since it is your thinking that makes you angry, you are responsible for feeling this way. Therefore, you are just as responsible for changing your thinking to help yourself to cope with anger, or at least to reduce it to a more manageable level.

- The best way to handle anger is probably to be in control so that it does not build up in the first place, to restructure your thinking so that your emotions do not get out of hand. But if anger does build up, remember that when it is channelled and used constructively, it can be beneficial. And when this is not possible, you can defuse or release your anger in a harmless way.

- **Let your anger out**. In general, one of the best outlets for releasing your anger is physical activity. Some people find that they can release the physical energy from anger by watching things – by, for example, watching a sporting event and really 'getting into' the activities you are viewing.

- Another common and very effective outlet for anger is crying. You have probably heard about the therapeutic effects of a good cry. If your anger has built up to the point of uncontrollable crying, this will be a great way to let it out!

- Some people like to count to ten when angry. This may distract you from what is making you angry, giving you a chance to calm down and think about it more constructively. Try counting out loud, and expressing your feelings through facial expressions and tone of voice.

Guilt

> **"**Sometimes I feel guilty about being a burden on my family especially if I have cheated a bit on my diet and that.**"**

> **"**I feel guilty because of being jealous and resentful of my friends and people, because they don't have diabetes and I do.**"**

Guilt is a very destructive emotion, one that can definitely interfere with your successful management of your diabetes, by lowering your self-image and exhausting your emotional resources. By becoming aware of how guilt develops, by pinpointing the source of your guilt, and by changing your thinking to be more positive and realistic, you should be able to decrease or eliminate this feeling, and instead use your energy to cope successfully with your condition.

Feelings of guilt usually have two components. The first of these is the sense of wrongdoing, the feeling that you have either done something wrong or have not done something you should have done. The second is the feeling of 'badness' that results from the self-blame, and this is a real problem. When you feel bad about doing something wrong, this is normal and understandable. But when you start telling yourself that you are a bad person, guilt follows.

People with diabetes feel guilty for lots of reasons. Maybe you are concerned about something you did to contribute to the development of your diabetes. Perhaps you feel that if it was not for certain actions, or lack of actions, on your part, you would not be in this situation. You may also feel guilty because you believe that you are complicating things for your family and therefore you blame yourself. Obviously, guilt can be a destructive emotion. It can drain you physically and emotionally, and can undermine your efforts to cope successfully with your diabetes.

HELPFUL TIPS! HELPFUL TIPS! HELPFUL TIPS! HELPFUL

There are various ways of 'handling' guilt:

- In order to cope successfully with guilt, you must first focus on what led to the guilty feelings in the first place. Sometimes, just by pinpointing the source of this emotion you can greatly reduce or even eliminate it.
- It is very important to discuss how you feel about your condition with others who may be affected by it. Share your concerns, and try to figure out solutions to any problems that exist. Try to ▶

turn your thoughts around: is there anything you can do about the negative thoughts that lead to guilt, those thoughts that make you feel that you're a bad person? Changing the emphasis in your thinking will also help you to lessen the perceived gap between what is and what you feel 'should' be, which is what led to the guilty feelings in the first place.

- Sometimes, when we feel guilt, and have failed to cope with this destructive emotion, we act in negative ways to hide from our feelings. There may be a tendency to indulge in 'escape' behaviour, such as drinking too much alcohol or excessive eating. Instead of dealing with the feelings head-on, we push them away.

- The first step towards improvement is to look past the escape behaviour and identify what is causing the guilt. Then think about what can be done to rectify the problem. At the same time, try to eliminate the escape behaviour, recognising that this activity is not improving your diabetes in any way. If you have difficulty eliminating this behaviour by yourself, or indeed identifying the root of the problem, then definitely consider working with a supportive health-care professional. It is possible, of course, that there is no clear-cut way to eliminate the situation or feelings that have led to your guilt. In that case, it may be helpful to look for partial solutions. These may not be as desirable as complete solutions, but they can still help to reduce your guilt and make you feel better about yourself.

Stress

Most of us have more first-hand experience with stress than we care to think about! The term 'stress' means many things to many different people. One person may define stress as pressure, tension or an emotional response. Stress is a response that occurs in your body as a reaction to the demands of everyday life resulting in physiological and psychological changes in the body. Many things occur each day that require us to adapt. These might include noise, crowding, a bad relationship, job interviews or commuting to work. These are known as *stressors*. The changes that take place in your body when something, 'the stressor', provokes you are known as the *stress response*. We all know that stress can play a role in causing or exacerbating virtually any medical problem, and diabetes is no exception. In fact, it has been suggested that any experience with diabetes both causes and can be affected by stress.

What are the symptoms of stress?

Physically, excessive stress can result in sweaty palms, heart palpitations, tightness of the throat, fatigue, nausea, diarrhoea or headaches. Emotionally, stress can manifest itself as depression, anxiety, anger, frustration, or simply as a vague feeling of uneasiness. The effects of stress are not isolated problems. Instead, they are part of a complex response that can affect both your body and your emotions.

How does stress affect the body?

Stress is a natural survival response. It occurs within the body when you feel threatened by thoughts or external stressors. When you are in a stressful situation, your circulatory system speeds up and blood is pushed rapidly towards different parts of the body, particularly those organs and systems necessary to protect you and this raises your blood pressure. Because the blood supply has been diverted, the supply to the digestive system is usually reduced as well, making the process of digestion slower and less effective. Stress also constricts the blood vessels, increases heart rate, and produces other physiological manifestations, all instantaneously!

You may also tremble or perspire. Your face may flush and you may feel a surge of adrenaline flowing through your body. Your mouth may become dry and you may feel nauseated. Your breathing may become more rapid and shallow. Your heart may begin to pound and your muscles may become tight, leading to headaches or cramps.

So, when you experience stress, your body prepares itself physiologically to counter any threat to its survival – the 'fight or flight' response. Stress may lead to physical problems: when you cannot respond in a way that eliminates it, the stress continues unabated and so do the symptoms. An inability to do anything to relieve the stress may cause even more stress, creating a vicious circle and this can take its toll on your body. In fact, many researchers believe that prolonged stress puts such a strain on your body that your immune system may ultimately break down, making your body more vulnerable to a number of diseases.

How does stress affect your diabetes?

Stress is particularly dangerous for people with diabetes. The hormones that the body releases as part of the fight or flight response are meant to prepare the body for quick action. These hormones break down stored glycogen into blood glucose, which the body should be able to use for energy. But people with diabetes cannot effectively use this extra glucose for energy, so the result is a rapid rise in blood sugar.

During times of stress, your self-care skills may also slip a little bit. When you're under pressure, for example if you have to meet a tight deadline, you may not take time to eat. Even if you do eat, the chances are that you won't spend too much time choosing foods that fit into your diet plan. Alternatively, maybe you'll decide to forgo exercise, because there are just too many other important things on your 'to do' list, or you may decide, like a number of people, to have a few 'drinks' or smoke a bit more to help you to relax when you're feeling stressed. Any of these behaviours can seriously affect your blood sugar levels.

Emotional response to stress

❝What people didn't see, and what I couldn't admit to, was the anxiety I felt if my blood glucose was the smallest amount above normal, and the desperation, the real stress I would feel until it had reduced.❞

Your emotional response to stress may not be as visible as your physical response. You may start worrying and fear the next 'event'. Your attention span may be reduced, and you may be less able to concentrate on the task at hand. You may have trouble learning something new. You may be afraid to do things and may withdraw or feel nervous. You may lose confidence in yourself.

As you become nervous and upset, you may become more aware of any unpleasant physical responses you are experiencing, and this may make you feel even more stressed. For example, if you have responded to stress with shallow, rapid breathing or heart palpitations, your awareness of these physical responses may lead to feelings of panic. Most people respond to stress both physically and emotionally, although it is possible to respond in only one way.

Is stress good or bad?

Stress can, of course, be either good or bad. It is good when it gives you extra energy to do the things that need to be done during stressful times. In fact, research suggests that a certain amount of stress is normal and necessary. Stress helps you to 'get your act together' and prepares you to handle your life in the best possible way. But when left unchecked, stress can be highly destructive, draining all of your energy and possibly worsening any existing physical or emotional problems.

What causes stress in diabetes?

A number of things can act as stressors. Work-related problems, marital disputes, family deaths, even some positive events, all of these can cause stress. Your diabetes can cause stress in a number of different ways. You may feel under a great deal of pressure to maintain 'perfect' control of your diabetes. You may feel stressed because the side-effects of diabetes are interfering with your sex life and relationships. Problems with your treatment or adjustments to dietary and lifestyle changes can cause stress. Fears of short- or long-term complications are also common stressors for people with diabetes, and indeed worries about being able to fulfil responsibilities may also provoke a stress response.

We all have a unique way of responding and your particular pattern of response to stress will depend on a number of things. Your upbringing, your self-esteem, your beliefs about yourself and the world, the way in which you guide yourself in your thoughts and actions – all of these things help to determine your stress response. The degree to which you feel in control of your life also plays an important role in this response, as does the way you feel, both physically and emotionally, and the way you get along with other people.

In summary, everyone's method of dealing with stress is unique and individual, and depends on a complex combination of thoughts and behaviours. Recent research suggests that stress is best understood as an interaction between each individual and his or her outside world, how each of us interprets and appraises events. It is the interaction of the stressor and our internal interpretation that determines the response to stress. This has important implications for coping with stress. It shows that stress is not solely the result of your environment, your illness, or any other factor around you. *The way you interpret the stressor is of equal importance.* In many situations, then, you do have the ability to control your reaction to the stressor.

How can you cope with stress?

Since stress can affect the body and mind in so many ways, stress management is a very important part of any programme for coping with diabetes. It is clear that stress can affect certain aspects of diabetes, including blood sugar levels. Importantly, you can learn effective strategies that will help you to deal with it. Obviously smoking, alcohol abuse, the use of inappropriate drugs, and overeating are all common but poor coping strategies. True, these activities will distract you and perhaps delay the effects of the stress, but they can also hurt you and prevent you from coping with stress in a constructive way. So, what should you do?

Relaxation techniques and regular exercise can be helpful parts of stress-management programmes. Also, by thinking more appropriate and positive thoughts, you can go a long way towards reducing stress as well. But be realistic and remember that while stress can be managed and controlled, it cannot be eliminated. Your focus, then, should be on using the following 'Helpful tips' to help you to deal better with both the physical and the emotional effects of the stress response.

HELPFUL TIPS! HELPFUL TIPS! HELPFUL TIPS! HELPFUL

There are various ways of 'handling' stress:

- **Relaxation benefits you in many ways**. First, it can give your body a chance to rest and recuperate. Also, a stronger body can help you to deal better with stress and life in general. Relaxation will help you sleep better, is pleasurable and will increase your feeling of emotional well-being. It can also give you a powerful sense of re-establishing control over your life, despite the presence of a chronic medical problem like diabetes. There are many different types of clinical relaxation techniques, including meditation and deep breathing, hypnosis and bio-feedback (discuss the technique that would be most appropriate for you with your diabetes team). One technique that is often successful in combating stress is imagery, which is the process of formulating mental pictures or scenes in order to harness your body's energy and improve your physical or emotional well-being. In this case, of course, you will want to conjure up images that are relaxing and stress-free. Imagine not only the sights but also the smell, the sensations and the sounds. The more vivid your image, the more helpful it will be. Feel comfortable with whatever degree of clarity your image takes on. The degree of relaxation you'll experience is up to you, and will benefit only you – you are in control.

- **Pinpoint the source of your stress**. Try to objectively identify your stressors and pinpoint what specifically is causing you to feel stress. Maybe you are having a hard time with the symptoms of diabetes. Maybe you are tired of sticking to your treatment programme, or maybe you are just tired of thinking about diabetes. There are many possibilities.

- **Identify your stress reactions**. Once you have begun identifying your stressors, you will want to become completely aware of your responses to them. Are they more physiological or psychological? What parts of your body seem to be the most vulnerable? What kinds of reaction does your body have? As you become more aware of these things, you will develop a complete picture of your own unique stress response. This

▶

picture will help you to choose the coping strategies that will be most useful in dealing with your stressors.

- **Eliminate stressors when possible**. Once you recognise the stressors that are causing the most trouble, try to determine whether you can eliminate them. Removing the source of stress is an obvious and logical way to manage it. For instance, if the task of managing your household expenses is causing you stress, you might talk to your partner and get that person to take over this task. Obviously, different types of stressors would have to be removed in different ways.

- **Change your view of the stressor**. What happens if you cannot eliminate the source of your stress, as is often the case? Then, the trick is to work on your interpretation of the stressors, using some of the techniques already discussed in 'Thinking Traps' on page 36.

- **Use physical activity to relieve stress**. Certain physical activities can be a great means of stress control. Exercise is not only a good way to release stress but can also be a very beneficial part of your diabetes treatment. Regardless of how diabetes is affecting you, there is certain to be a type of exercise that will help you to control your level of stress. Brisk walking, swimming and dancing, for instance, all allow for the release of tension. Obviously you should get your doctor's approval before beginning any increased physical activity programme.

- **Use hobbies and other leisure activities to reduce stress**. These activities are often very effective as they can divert your attention from the stressful situation and direct it towards something more enjoyable. They may also help you to feel more productive, and a lack of a feeling of productivity may be one of the stressors giving you problems in the first place! If you don't have a hobby, this may be the time to investigate something that has always interested you. If you are already involved in a hobby, you now have the perfect reason to indulge yourself whenever you can.

❝One of the good things about having diabetes is that it makes a virtue out of enjoying myself. The little 'doctor' in the back of my head smiles when I go dancing or swimming, my prescription includes having fun. **99**

- **Catch up on your sleep**. Some people have difficulty sleeping when they are experiencing high levels of stress. But, when possible, prolonged periods of sleep may help you to reduce your stress to a more manageable level.

Fears

When you were first diagnosed, many fearful questions probably came to mind. *'What will the future be like? What will become of me?'*

These are typical questions of people who are diagnosed with any chronic medical problem, not just diabetes. As time goes by, some of these initial questions will have been answered and you will have started to adjust to your life with diabetes. But once your initial fears are reduced, new fears may arise focusing on more specific questions. You may now start to be afraid that you will not manage your self-care, or fear that you may develop long-term complications or other events and experiences. All of these fears are usual and understandable, and should be expected, but however 'normal' they may be, they can become extremely harmful if you fail to cope with them effectively.

Fear of needles, for example, is very common, even for people who do not have diabetes. Some people delay going to the doctor, because their dislike of needles is so intense, but if you need insulin, avoiding the use of needles is just not an option.

The good news is that most people who take insulin report that the anticipation of taking insulin injections is much worse than the actual injections. Additionally, your diabetes team will be there to guide you as you learn to give yourself injections, and they will teach you safe and efficient ways to inject your insulin so that the process will be as smooth and as quick as possible. There is also specialist help available, if necessary, to help you to deal with your fear of needles and injections.

Fear of developing complications is also very common among people with diabetes, which is totally understandable. Lots of people with diabetes are afraid they will have to restrict their activities because of physical problems such as neuropathy or retinopathy. Many fear that they will be disabled because of diabetes-related complications.

HELPFUL TIPS! HELPFUL TIPS! HELPFUL TIPS! HELPFUL

There are various ways of 'handling' fear:

- One solution is to tell yourself that having diabetes does not mean that complications are inevitable; even if they do occur, the effects may not be severe, and you are not going to develop complications just because you *think* it might happen! Fear can actually be a good motivator. If you are afraid of developing complications, perhaps you will be more inspired to take good care of yourself and control your diabetes to the best of your ability.

- If you are finding that diabetes has placed some restrictions on your activities, you may be afraid of becoming too dependent on your friends and family. You may worry that you will be too much of a burden on your loved ones if you ask for help and fear that you will lose your ability to help yourself. Dealing with this fear is helped by concentrating on those things that you still can do. Graciously accept the help you may have to take from others, but do not view this as dependence. Instead, focus on the benefits you are receiving from increased interaction with family and friends.

- Nobody likes pain, and you may be fearful of the pain that may develop as a result of a diabetes-related complication. Each little twinge of pain may make you afraid that a more serious problem is developing, and even when you are not in pain, you may fear its occurrence. Try to accept the fact that you will experience some pain from time to time, but that medication can reduce its intensity as well as its duration.

- Are you afraid of the reactions of other people when they know you have diabetes? Many people feel that there is a 'stigma' attached to having diabetes, and that people might shy away from you if they knew. Unfortunately, some people can be cold and unfeeling and may be put off by the fact that you have to use injections or that you can no longer keep up with them.

- Remember that your true friends will accept you in any circumstances. Of course, if you feel that an important relationship is in jeopardy, you should try to figure out why, and what you can do to improve things, and if you feel that people are shying away from you, try to discuss this with them. You may be able to remedy the situation, or get appropriate counselling if necessary, but it is also important to remember that you can only do so much and if your efforts do not work, at least you will know that you did your best. You may find it helpful to get involved in a support group where you will know that people are going through the same things as you and may even be able to give you some tips, because of their own experiences, on dealing with family and friends.

❝I didn't think anyone could understand what I was up against, until I went, not very willingly, to a diabetes support group. For the first time I got to talk to people who were struggling with the same issues that had me down. They taught me an awful lot about things I could do to help myself.**❞**

- Like many people with diabetes you may be concerned about the effect your condition will have on your job and worry about how long your employer will continue to be tolerant and understanding. Of course, your need for money may also be greater due to your medical problems so the pressure can be tremendous. Again, talk to others who have been in the same situation, and see how they handled it and, if necessary, speak to experts who can advise you on financial matters. Your diabetes team will be able to discuss these issues with you.

- Travelling with diabetes can present special challenges and circumstances. To some people with diabetes, the preparation required to take a 'relaxing' holiday can be overwhelming, and the thought of travelling far from familiar medical facilities can be very frightening. However, proper planning can ensure that you have a safe and enjoyable holiday. Always take more than enough medication with you just in case your return home is delayed. Carry your medication and other supplies with you at all times so that they are readily available if you need them and, of course, research your destination before you go to find out how to get medical care. Your travel agent will help you.

- Many individuals with diabetes have a significant fear of not coping. You may feel that you are barely handling your diabetes and believe that any new problem that comes along will be enough to push you over the edge. This fear can easily lead to ▶

panic, so it is important to pinpoint those particular problems and get help to deal with them. Do not wait, and do not project a false sense of bravado. If you feel that you are nearing the edge, get someone to help you to steady yourself. Talk over your fears with someone. Once you have shared them, you may see things a little more clearly. You may be able to deal with problems with greater strength, knowing that you are not alone.

Although many different fears have been discussed in this section, all of the fears that you have experienced have probably not been covered. In addition, the coping suggestions offered certainly do not include all possible ways of dealing with fear.

Anticipate that you will be fearful of certain things from time to time. Some fears will return, but try to 'ride' them rather than succumbing to them. Remember it is perfectly normal to be afraid! The most important thing is to stay on top of those fears to ensure that they do not overwhelm you or render you less able to cope. Therefore, work on recognising your fears. For some of them, you will modify your behaviour; for others, you will modify your thinking. This will help you to feel more in control and, as this happens, you will notice that your fears begin to diminish. That does not mean that they will all go away, but as you work on them, they will at least lessen in intensity and you will feel better knowing that you can handle whatever comes along.

Summary

- The diagnosis of diabetes can have a tremendous psychological impact on each individual.

- How people attempt to make sense of the diagnosis and try to understand the implications of having diabetes will depend on their beliefs about the illness. Two beliefs in particular are thought to relate to long-term adjustment: beliefs about the cause of the illness ('Why did it happen?') and beliefs about whether or not it can be cured or controlled ('What can I do to manage it now?').

- Some of the common reactions to diagnosis include denial, anxiety, relief, depression, anger and stress.

- Lower psychological distress is associated with positive, confrontative coping responses and with beliefs that one can personally direct control over the illness.

- Increasing physical activity and restructuring thinking patterns are key elements in coping with these common emotional reactions.

What about interacting with other people?

4

This chapter will discuss interacting with other people, not just family, friends and colleagues, but also the many health-care professionals involved in your diabetes care.

❝Having diabetes is not exactly something you want to shout from the roof tops, in fact you can feel like hiding it completely. But there are some people who need to know and others who can support you more if they do.**❞**

You interact with many people every day and you will certainly want to be able to deal with any difficulties you are likely to have in your interpersonal relationships. You might worry about what others are going to think now that you have been diagnosed with diabetes and how they might react. Obviously, different problems exist in different relationships, and in this chapter we discuss how to get the best from your consultations, coping with comments people make, living with someone who has diabetes and, importantly, dealing with children with diabetes.

What about my family?

Family and friends will probably be among the first people you tell about your diabetes and they can be an important source of emotional support and practical assistance as you learn to cope with your problem. Like most people, they will probably know little about it, but as they will probably be keen to learn more you may find yourself teaching them about diabetes. You may also find yourself on the receiving end of sketchy stories about someone's great aunt 'who had a touch of sugar'. One topic that will almost certainly be discussed is diet. Your partner or family will want to know what you can eat and how it will affect them; but because the recommended diet is in fact the same healthy diet that can be followed by everyone, they will not have to make any special arrangements for you. They might also like to start eating more healthily anyway, to keep you company!

Diabetes may create the need for changes in each family member's responsibilities, as your partner or children take over some of the functions that you performed in the past. This can be a potential source of friction within the family, especially if some people feel that they are now taking on a heavier share of the load. It is therefore important to discuss the needed changes with them and make any changes gradually, trying to avoid overwhelming your family. You should also be realistic in your expectations and remember that it takes time for anyone to comfortably incorporate new responsibilities into their routines. Children, regardless of how old they are, may be especially vulnerable to the stresses and strains that occur when a family member has a chronic illness. You can help your children to handle any fears or changes that may be troubling them by encouraging them to ask questions and by trying to give direct answers, or further information as and when they ask for it.

What about my friends and colleagues?

Before your diagnosis, your relationships with your friends may have been fairly effortless. Unfortunately, diabetes can change that. You may be surprised or hurt by the seeming aloofness of some friends, while others may be too supportive. Then, of course, there are the special problems that may crop up because of your condition, such as the need to ask for help. These problems can sometimes take a toll on seemingly strong friendships.

How can you deal with this? Because your friends and colleagues have not been directly affected by it, they may not be able to understand fully what you are experiencing. Some may want to learn more; some may want to forget what little they already know. You should certainly be prepared for a variety of reactions to your diabetes. Some friends, for instance, may seem uninterested and distant, perhaps because they feel that they just do not know what to say to you. Their doubts and fears may cause so much tension that they may not even want to be with you. Others, of course, may be very supportive – perhaps too supportive! There may be times when friends and colleagues are constantly asking you how you are or offering help when you would rather be left alone. Certainly, friendships can suffer because of misunderstandings and uncertainties, so, in the beginning, try to establish some ground rules. If you are the kind of person who likes to be asked how you feel, then let your friends know. If you would rather not be asked, then let your friends know that too. Your changing feelings may be difficult for friends and colleagues to deal with so let them know that they can talk to you whenever they want to and you will let them know if you are having trouble coping. If you clear up most of the 'question marks', fewer unknowns will exist and the uneasiness about what to do or say, which can often affect relationships, will be reduced.

What about the health-care professionals?

The quality of the relationship between you and the health-care professionals involved in your care will in large part determine your perception of the quality of the care itself. Relationships characterised by respect, trust and genuine caring facilitate open and honest communication between both parties. You will feel psychologically safe enough to explore and express your deepest fears and concerns related to having diabetes. Also, in a relationship characterised by trust and respect, you are much more likely to value the suggestions and recommendations of the health-care professionals.

Establishing such relationships requires effort and commitment. A great many factors will determine your ability to feel comfortable with your health-care team including your personality, your health-care professionals' personality and philosophy regarding treatment, and more. You will probably look for a series of cues in order to answer important questions that you will have on your mind, such as 'Do they listen to me?', 'Do they seem to care about people?', 'Are they concerned about my agenda and my concerns?', 'Do they appear knowledgeable about diabetes?', 'Will they be able to answer my questions?'.

How these questions are answered will determine the extent to which you will feel that you can be open and candid with the diabetes team and take heed of their recommendations.

Partnership

In the case of diabetes, both the health-care professionals and the patient have expertise that is equally important to the development of a sound diabetes treatment programme. The health-care professionals know about diabetes and understand the various management options and their potential health-related consequences. You are an expert on your own life and in the best position to decide which of the various diabetes care approaches is realistic for you. Because diabetes involves such sweeping changes in your lifestyle, your own self-awareness is crucial to the development of an effective treatment programme. The fact that each person in the patient–health-care professionals relationship brings expertise of equal importance makes a true partnership possible. However, for the diabetes–care partnership to work, both parties have to recognise and respect the expertise of the other. This kind of collaboration is quite unique to diabetes care and is a significant departure from the usual consultation style.

The consultation

Most of your communications with the health-care professionals will take place during your visits to the diabetes clinic and you should aim to make these visits as helpful and as productive as possible. We have all come away from a visit to the doctor at one stage or another and realised that we forgot to ask an important question, and this can be very frustrating. The following 'Helpful tips' provide a number of things you can do to help you to get the most out of your visits to the health-care professionals involved in your care.

HELPFUL TIPS! HELPFUL TIPS! HELPFUL TIPS! HELPFUL

There are various ways of 'handling' a consultation:

- **Make a list**. Before each appointment, it is important to prepare a list of all the questions you want to ask the doctor. Prepare this list by jotting down notes whenever you think of a question or piece of information or something you do not understand about your diabetes. Many people worry that the questions they wish to ask are too trivial or silly, but if you need further information about any aspect of your treatment or condition, then you must feel free to ask. This will make it easier for the health-care professionals to respond with the kind of information that you actually need.

- **Getting the answers**. As your questions are answered, be sure to listen carefully. If you are worried that you will not remember everything that occurs or is said to you then you can either jot down the answers to your questions or bring a family member or close friend with you for the clinic visit. It can be very helpful to bring someone with you when you visit the doctor or other health-care professional. It is so easy to miss what is being said sometimes, especially if you are tense or anxious about the visit. So having another 'set of ears' will increase the likelihood that all the important information will be retained. It may also remove some of your pressure, and help you to relax and get the most out of the visit.

Satisfaction with treatment

It is very important to make sure that you understand what your health-care professionals are saying to you and to speak up when you do not understand because they are being either too vague or using medical 'jargon' or technical language with which you are not familiar. Good communication is critical if you are to be satisfied with your care, and a number of studies have linked 'satisfaction with treatment' to a good understanding of what was said during the consultation, which in turn leads to the likelihood of being able to follow your treatment recommendations. Poor communication between patients and health-care professionals, on the other hand, has been linked to dissatisfaction with the care you are receiving and to problems, such as not following your treatment recommendations and even not attending for future visits.

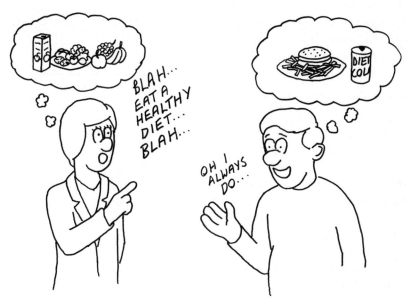

Health-care professionals and patients may not be speaking the same language

Negotiating goals

The main objective of any diabetes care programme is to provide a service that encourages partnership with you in any decisions that are made about your diabetes, supports you in managing your diabetes, and helps you to adopt and maintain a healthy lifestyle, so that you will have choice and control over what happens to you at each step of your care. An agreed, negotiated, shared care plan, with specific goals and objectives, set out in a format and language appropriate for you, is therefore essential to the achievement of this objective.

Setting goals has become more common in diabetes care as part of meeting the need for improved standards of care. Goal setting can be seen as a way of identifying choices for an individual rather than imposing expectations. Whenever we make significant changes in our lives, we give up some things (costs) and gain others (benefits). We make changes when the benefits of solving a problem outweigh the costs of changing our behaviour. The decision that a particular goal is appropriate to help to solve a problem can only be made by the person with the problem.

Box 4.	Considering the costs and benefits of change.

	Benefits of change	Costs of change
For me		
For those around me		
My reactions		
The reactions of others		

If goal setting is to succeed, therefore, the goals need to flow from you and be an expression of what you require to solve a particular problem. The goals need to come from you and be owned by you. This can be particularly challenging, as people sometimes want to set goals that are far too ambitious to be achievable. In other circumstances people want to set goals that are not compatible with established guidelines or with what the diabetes care team believe is the best course. However, your health-care professionals will ensure that you understand the disadvantages and benefits of your decisions, and will emphasise the likely consequences of your choices. In the end, however, you are responsible for, and in control of, the choices you make about your own diabetes self-care.

HELPFUL TIPS! HELPFUL TIPS! HELPFUL TIPS! HELPFUL

One approach to helping people to set realistic goals in diabetes care is based on the acronym SMART – that is, goals must be **S**pecific, **M**easurable, **A**greed, **R**ealistic and **T**ime-specific.

A 'SMART' goal-setting plan should be:

- **Specific**. The goal needs to be specific, so rather than saying 'I am going to eat healthily', you need to specify exactly what you are going to do, e.g. 'I am going to buy low-fat crisps'.

- **Measurable**. It should be possible to monitor or gauge the task when you have done it. This is easier if the goal is specific because then you will know whether you have achieved it or not.

- **Agreed**. The specific goal is not 'forced' upon you by health-care professionals or others involved in your care. It is negotiated and agreed between you.

▶

- **Realistic**. The goal must be realistically achievable by you. It is important that progress is made in small achievable steps, which will build your self-confidence and increase your motivation to continue.
- **Time-specific**. As it is very important that you know when you have achieved your goal, there must be a clear agreement about when you are going to do it, how long for, how often and when progress will be reviewed.

What about comments from others?

66How can you stand giving yourself injections? Do you feel like a pincushion or a bit of a junky?99

66Is diabetes contagious?99

66You must miss the way you used to feel.99

66I certainly don't envy you.99

66If you ate right, you would feel a lot better.99

'You look awful!'

It can be very upsetting when somebody says this. You may be feeling awful but you probably do not want to be reminded of it. Even if it is said sympathetically, you may find this kind of remark insulting.

'What is diabetes?'

Some people really do not understand what diabetes is all about, and they will bluntly ask you to explain your condition. This kind of question usually does show some genuine concern, so in some circumstances you might want to explain just a little more about what diabetes is and how it affects you. But if this is the twentieth time that you have heard that question, it may be difficult to respond cheerfully. In fact, many people feel that there is a stigma attached to having diabetes.

Legitimate comments

Many of the things people say to you may be legitimate comments with sincere concern for your health, but they may be extremely irritating to you just the same. Other remarks may be made without any consideration for your feelings whatsoever. It doesn't really matter why a comment is inappropriate; the important thing is that you learn to cope with some of the comments you hear in a way that is comfortable for you.

HELPFUL TIPS! HELPFUL TIPS! HELPFUL TIPS! HELPFUL

There are various ways of 'handling' questions and comments from others:

- One way is to simply ignore the comment. This is not always easy, especially if the person persistently waits for your answer or seems genuinely insulted by your lack of response.

- Another way of responding to irritating comments is to answer in a rational and intelligent way, explaining how you feel or what you sincerely want to communicate. This may be sufficient to stop some people making remarks or asking questions. However, you may not always be able to cope by ignoring a remark or responding to it rationally, and what can you do then?

- A third possibility is to respond to comments humorously, letting the person know that the remark was inappropriate. In this way you can also have a bit of fun without saying things that you might later regret! As you now know, you cannot change other people. You cannot make them more sensitive or teach them how to be more tactful but you can learn to cope in a way that is comfortable for you, and as you learn to respond more comfortably to these comments you will find that you can cope with them more calmly.

What about living with someone who has diabetes?

A chronic medical condition like diabetes does not just affect the sufferer; it also affects everyone close to that person. In fact, those who are closest are likely to be the most profoundly affected, but they are also in the best position to help.

Illness can create a number of changes in any relationship, and not always for the better. If you live with someone who has diabetes, you may now see that person, and even yourself, differently. Maybe you see the person with diabetes as being more fragile. You may even feel guilty about that person's condition, or about your feelings regarding his or her condition. Maybe you were quite dependent on that person and now you have to shoulder more responsibility.

If you are close to someone with diabetes, you can help enormously by learning as much as you can about the condition and its treatment. This will enable you to provide support and true understanding. Knowing the facts may also help you to conquer your fears of the unknown and eliminate your confusion over symptoms, treatments, and side-effects.

You can also show your support by participating in some aspects of his or her treatment. For example, you can be an exercise 'buddy' or change your eating patterns so that the person with diabetes will not feel 'different' and a burden on the relationship or that he or she is depriving you of tasty foods.

Living with diabetes can be difficult. You may sympathise and this may help you to provide beneficial support. Going overboard with 'pity' can, however, be destructive. Your goal is to try to make life as normal as possible for the person with diabetes. Do not assume that you must be overprotective or underprotective simply because that is the way you would want others to act if you were ill. Be sure to find out what the person with diabetes needs, and try to act accordingly. The key to maintaining harmony is good communication.

Take care of yourself, too! You can't be strong for others if you don't take care of yourself as well. It is true that the diabetes is not affecting your body, but it is certainly affecting you in other ways. You may experience many of the same emotions and changes in lifestyle experienced by the person with diabetes, but feel more helpless because everything is happening *around* you rather than *to* you. So remember to take some time out for yourself, and when you are refreshed you will be all the more ready to help the person who has diabetes to cope with the condition.

What about children with diabetes?

&&I was absolutely devastated when my son was diagnosed with diabetes, I thought 'Oh no, why couldn't it have been me not him?', the feelings of guilt, anger, and grief even, were overwhelming, it was as though I had lost my 'healthy' child and he had been replaced with this other one.&&

Children and young people with diabetes are subject to all the normal pressures and pleasures of physical, emotional and social development. Their needs as individuals within a family or family system, and the role of their parents or carers and siblings in sustaining them from initial diagnosis through childhood to independence, are essential.

When a child is diagnosed with diabetes, the critical tasks of decision making concerning the child's daily survival and treatment are transferred from health-care professionals to the family. Immediately following diagnosis, the family is responsible for carefully balancing multiple daily insulin injections and food intake with physical activity in order to prevent large fluctuations in blood glucose levels, which can interfere with the child's normal growth and development. Frequent blood glucose monitoring is also required to assess this fine balance between insulin, food and activity. It is well documented that this complex daily regimen impacts on every aspect of the child's development and family life, and that good emotional adjustment is strongly related to better glucose control.

It is very common for parents and families to have trouble coping with a child's illness and therefore good rapport and communication with the health-care professionals involved in your child's diabetes care is essential. Support groups and educational materials targeted towards families of very young children can help parents and families to feel less alone and can normalise feelings of guilt, anxiety and fear. It is important to accept the fact that diabetes won't just 'go away', but remember that diabetes management must not take over your family's life. Love, guide and discipline your child as if diabetes were not a factor and tell yourself that a diagnosis of diabetes does not have to be totally negative; people grow and change not only when things are going well, but also when they are not!

Because the school environment presents many opportunities for building self-esteem and developing socialisation skills, it is important for the child with diabetes to participate fully in all activities, with as few restrictions as possible, in order to facilitate a normal school experience. Children need to understand that, although they have diabetes, they are not 'sick' or 'abnormal'. Participation in school activities helps to minimise the child's sense of being different from peers. Some modifications in a typical school day may need to be made to accommodate diabetes safely, such as the scheduling of lunch and gym classes, but restricting the child from gym classes or school outings will only emphasise the 'difference' and may foster a sense of inferiority and lack of confidence.

One area of importance for families and health-care professionals concerns issues of transferring diabetes care responsibilities from the parent to the child. Findings from a number of recent important studies suggest that children and adolescents given greater responsibility for their diabetic management make more mistakes in their self-care, and have poorer blood glucose control than those whose parents are more involved. From these studies it has become increasingly clear that parental involvement in diabetes management is required throughout the school-age developmental period. Each family needs to negotiate its own acceptable pattern of parent–child teamwork, based on factors such as the child's temperament and your availability. By identifying *'shared responsibility'* rather than *'child independence'* as the expectation, the health-care team can help make parent involvement seem less inappropriate to the child. The clear message is that diabetes management tasks must be 'protected' from the child's normal drive to achieve independent mastery.

HELPFUL TIPS! HELPFUL TIPS! HELPFUL TIPS! HELPFUL

There are various ways of 'handling' parental pitfalls:

- **Over-indulgence**. Some parents believe that the rigors of self-care are too intense for their child to handle, so they offer special treats while providing little discipline. As a result, the child learns poor self-care skills, and may feel incapable of handling self-care when the time comes.

- **Over-protection**. In this case, the parents are so worried about their child's health that they continue to handle most of the details of diabetes management, even when their child is old enough to assume responsibility for treatment. A child raised in this type of environment tends to be over-dependent, lacking the self-confidence necessary to be fully responsible for self-care.

- **Indifference**. Indifferent parents are the opposite extreme, they do not fuss enough over their child's care, and do not provide the necessary discipline and supportive environment that the child needs to learn good self-care skills. The danger here is that the child may 'rebel' and seek attention through negative behaviours, such as skipping insulin injections, 'forgetting' to do blood glucose tests, or eating the wrong foods. Obviously, these behaviours can have some very serious physical effects.

Summary

- You interact with many people every day and you will want to be able to deal with any difficulties you are likely to have in your interpersonal relationships as a result of your diabetes.

- Family and friends will probably be among the first people you tell about having diabetes and they can be an important source of emotional support and practical assistance as you learn to cope with your diabetes.

- The quality of the relationship between you and the health-care professionals involved in your care will, in large part, determine your perception of the quality of the care itself.

- In a relationship characterised by trust and respect, you are much more likely to value the suggestions and recommendations of the health-care professionals.

- Good communication between you and the health-care professionals is critical if you are to be satisfied with your care, and a number of studies have linked 'satisfaction with treatment' to a good understanding and remembering of what was being said during the consultation.

- If you live with someone who has diabetes you can help enormously by learning as much as possible about the condition and its treatment.

- When a child is diagnosed with diabetes, the critical tasks of decision making concerning the child's daily survival and treatment are transferred from health-care professionals to the family.

- The complex daily regimen impacts on every aspect of the child's development and family life, and good emotional adjustment for the child is strongly related to better glucose control.

Understanding and managing treatment

5

Although at present diabetes cannot be cured, it can be treated very successfully. Treatment for diabetes varies from person to person and will depend on the type of diabetes you have.

66Years ago it was really restrictive having diabetes, but I think there is a greater understanding now, not so restrictive as before, things are more easily related to every day life. 99

66Diabetes is not such a problem now because you can control it, I feel that insulin kinda takes away the diabetes. 99

66I felt so ill on tablets but now I'm on insulin and things are much better.99

This chapter will focus on understanding and managing the different types of treatment available, including medication, healthy eating, increasing physical activity levels, and discuss the goals that people with diabetes should aim for when they undertake treatment.

Understanding and managing treatment with medication

Type 1 diabetes is treated by injections of insulin and a healthy diet, and regular exercise is recommended. Type 2 diabetes is treated by a healthy diet and exercise or by a combination of a healthy diet, exercise and tablets. Eventually people with type 2 diabetes may also need insulin injections, although they are not totally 'dependent' on the insulin. If you have just been diagnosed as type 2, it is bound to take you some time to adjust to the idea, but with the right information and back-up from your diabetes care team, you will soon realise that you will be able to cope and keep yourself well. They will show you how to give injections, and take time to teach you how to manage your condition effectively. Do not worry if you need to see them several times to clarify certain points, no one will mind, and would prefer you to ask questions and come back until you feel comfortable with all the new information you have to cope with.

Tablets

There are four main kinds of tablet treatment for people with type 2 diabetes: sulphonylureas, biguanides, acarbose and thiazolidinediones. They all come under the general name of *oral hypoglycaemic agents* (OHAs), and any of them may be taken alone or in combination. Many people with type 2 diabetes find that these medications, together with a healthy eating pattern, keep their diabetes under control, although it may take some time to find out which combination or dose suits you best.

The tablets all work in different ways: some help your pancreas to produce more insulin; others help your body to make better use of the insulin that your pancreas does produce; and yet others slow down the speed at which your body absorbs glucose from the intestine. Your doctor will decide which kinds of tablet are going to work best for you and may prescribe more than one kind. Your doctor or diabetes nurse will tell you all about the tablets, when to take them, and how to monitor your blood or urine glucose levels.

> **❝**Going on to insulin, I found this really upsetting – felt I was doing well and it was a reflection on me to say going on to insulin.**❞**

Eventually even several types of tablet may not be enough to keep your blood glucose levels within the normal range and you may be advised to take insulin as well as, or instead of, your tablets. This is quite a usual thing to happen and is not a reflection on you or on how well you have been looking after yourself.

Insulin

People with type 1 diabetes need injections of insulin for the rest of their lives and also need to eat a healthy diet that contains the right balance of foods. In addition, a minimum of exercise is recommended for overall health and to prevent diabetes complications.

'Why do I have to inject the insulin?'

This is the only effective way of getting it into your bloodstream. Insulin cannot be swallowed because the digestive juices in the stomach destroy it.

'What types of insulin are there?'

The basic difference is in how quickly they take effect, so they can be divided into short-, medium- or long-acting varieties. The short-acting insulin is always clear or colourless, whereas the other two are cloudy because they contain additives to slow down the absorption of insulin from under the skin. It is possible to mix short- and medium-acting insulin in the same syringe, but care must be taken not to contaminate the clear insulin with any cloudy insulin. For this reason the clear insulin is always drawn up first.

If you find it difficult to mix the insulin yourself, you may be able to use one of the ready-mixed kinds which contain short- and medium-acting insulin in different proportions.

All three types of insulin may be produced from animal sources – pig or beef – or from genetically engineered human hormone. Some so-called human insulin is in fact derived originally from pigs but altered so that it is indistinguishable from the human version. The human type is the most widely prescribed insulin in the UK.

'Why do I have to inject insulin several times a day?'

The object of insulin therapy is to imitate the body's natural supply of insulin as closely as possible. In a person who does not have diabetes, insulin is released by the pancreas in response to food. As the blood glucose level falls between meals, so the insulin level drops back towards zero. It never quite gets there, however, and there is no time in the 24 hours when there is no detectable insulin in the bloodstream. What you are trying to do when you give yourself insulin injections is to reproduce the normal pattern of insulin production from the pancreas.

There are several ways of doing this using different types of insulin and numbers of injections per day. For example, many people follow a system which comprises three injections of short-acting insulin before the three main meals of the day, plus a night-time injection of a medium- or long-acting insulin to control blood glucose while they are asleep. Another popular and equally successful system involves two injections a day of a mixture of short- and medium-acting insulin. The idea is that the short-acting component covers the meal you are about to have – for example, breakfast or the evening meal – while the medium-acting component covers you at lunchtime or overnight. Many people have been using one or other of these systems very happily for years, and the choice between them is often simply a matter of personal preference.

If you are one of the relatively few people who simply cannot get used to giving yourself several injections a day, or if you have only a partial failure of your insulin supply, you may be able to make do with just one or two daily injections of medium- or long-acting insulin.

'How and where do I inject myself?'

Your diabetes care team will show you how to do the injections and explain the various types of equipment available. Many people today use disposable plastic syringes and needles. Insulin injection pens are also very popular, largely because of their convenience and portability. Although the pens themselves are free, the needles still have to be paid for, although there is currently an active campaign to try to persuade the Department of Health to allow free prescription of pen needles. There are several types of pen to choose from, but the principles of the device are much the same. It is simply a matter of which one suits you best.

You inject insulin under your skin rather than into a vein or muscle. Recent research has suggested that many people may have been getting the depth wrong so that insulin is going into the muscle beneath the skin by mistake. Judging the depth accurately can be a problem, especially if you are slim, but it is important to master the technique because insulin can be absorbed from muscle more rapidly than expected. Your diabetes care team will show you how to do it properly, but many people find that the simplest way is to pinch the skin and inject the bunched up area at an angle of 90 degrees. Don't pinch too hard, however, or it will hurt when the needle goes in! For people who may be having difficulty with inadvertent muscular injection, there are different lengths of needle available and this problem should be discussed with your diabetes care team.

You will be given advice about the best sites for injection. The tops of the thighs, buttocks and abdomen are the most common sites, and it is best to avoid using the same area every time, otherwise you could develop a small fatty lump, which could affect the smoothness of insulin absorption. It is probably a good idea to inject medium- or long-acting insulin into your thigh or buttock and use your tummy for short-acting injections, but the most important thing is that you should be reasonably comfortable about the sites you are using.

'Will the injections hurt or mark?'

People who have been giving themselves injections for years say they do not feel a thing, but many beginners may find it slightly painful at first. Try to be as relaxed as you can and follow the technique you have been shown. Some people find that it helps to rub the skin with ice for a few seconds beforehand to numb it, and you might like to try this method. As you get more practice, you should find that the injections rarely hurt, but if things do not improve, it is worth asking someone at the diabetes centre for advice on what is causing the problem.

The needles are very fine and usually do not leave a mark. Sometimes you may get a little bleeding after an injection or even a bruise, but this is nothing to worry about. It just means that you have probably punctured one of the tiny blood vessels

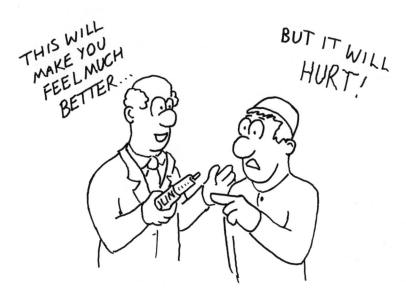

Fear of injections is very common

under the skin, which happens occasionally. There is virtually no chance of insulin directly entering the bloodstream, so do not worry if you notice some bleeding.

Box 5.	Key points about treatment with medication.

- Tablet treatment is useful for type 2 diabetes.
- Tablets work in different ways and have different effects.
- Insulin injections are necessary for all type 1 and many type 2 patients.
- At least two and maybe four injections are needed each day.
- Injections rarely cause discomfort or leave any mark.
- Insulin preparations can be short, medium or long acting.
- New pre-mixed short- and medium-acting preparations are now available.

Understanding and managing healthy eating

Why change what you eat?

What you eat has an effect on your general health and well-being. Many people think that they already have a healthy diet but, on average, people in the UK eat too much fat and too many calories. This can result in high cholesterol levels and weight problems and lead to many heart attacks each year.

Whichever type of diabetes you have, your food choice helps to balance your blood glucose levels and your diet is therefore an essential part of your treatment. However, the sort of diet you should follow when you have diabetes definitely does not mean a future of self-denial on all tasty foods. Changing your eating habits does not mean that you need to follow a special diet, but just a healthy diet as recommended for everyone.

> **❝**It's all changed now – makes a huge difference not to have to weigh every piece of food. Everything had to be counted before.**❞**

Eating more healthily can reduce your risk of developing:

- Complications of diabetes.
- Heart disease by reducing cholesterol levels, blood pressure, weight.
- Some cancers (two-thirds of cancer are related to what we eat).
- Arthritis.

To eat healthily, what are you aiming for?

> **❝**My friend's grandfather was diabetic. She said I should never touch starch. Fatal, you see, for a diabetic. Makes sugar. So I'm always very strict. No bread, no biscuits, no potato ever.**❞**

The *Balance of Good Health* (see Figure 2) shows the types and proportion of foods you need to eat to achieve a well-balanced and healthy diet. It is based on the five commonly accepted food groups. It shows that you do not have to give up the foods you most enjoy for the sake of your health. A healthy eating pattern includes the correct balance of foods from the four main food groups every day, plus an allowance for extras from the fats and fatty sugary foods group. All your nutritional needs will be met if you choose foods in these proportions. Remember, however, that everything you eat – snacks as well as meals – counts towards the balance of what you eat. The basic message is:

- **Base your meals on starchy foods – fill up on these**. This means such foods as bread, potatoes, rice, pasta, noodles, oats, crackers, breakfast cereals. These all provide starch, fibre, vitamins (especially B) and minerals.
- **Eat at least five servings of fruit and vegetables daily**. Choose from fresh, frozen, or canned fruit and vegetables – and do not forget juices and dried fruit. Add in some to each meal or snack from breakfast to bedtime. These contain

The balance of good health

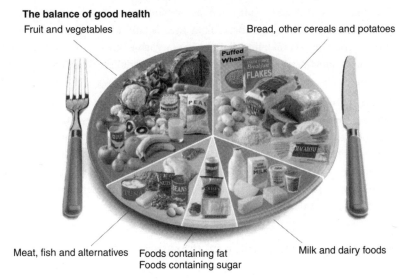

Fruit and vegetables

Bread, other cereals and potatoes

Meat, fish and alternatives

Foods containing fat
Foods containing sugar

Milk and dairy foods

Figure 2. The plate model. Reproduced by kind permission of the Food Standards Agency

vitamins, minerals and fibre. Eating them may help to protect you against heart disease and cancer as they contain antioxidant vitamins (vitamins A, C, and E).

- **Eat moderate amounts of milk and dairy foods, and lower fat versions whenever you can**. These contain calcium, protein and vitamins A and B.

- **Eat moderate amounts of meat, fish and alternatives and choose lower fat versions**. Lower fat choices include lean meat, chicken, fish, eggs, beans and pulses. These foods contain protein and iron. Try to have fish at least twice a week and use beans and pulses to make meat go further or for a meat-free meal.

- **Reduce your intake of fats and fatty and sugary foods**. Fats in the diet is the main problem as far as heart disease, high blood cholesterol and weight gain are concerned. *They are of limited nutritional value and you can obtain all the fat you need from the milk, dairy, meat and meat alternatives groups.* Use spreading fats and cooking oils sparingly. Keep fatty and sugary dishes and snacks as occasional rather than everyday foods. *Choose low fat methods of preparation and cooking.*

Intake of fats

Two main types of fat are normally consumed:

- **Saturated fats (or 'saturates')**. The more saturates we eat, the more cholesterol the body produces. This builds up in our blood and increases the risk of developing heart disease. Saturated fats are found mostly in animal products such as dairy products and meat. They are also found in some vegetable oils such as coconut oil and palm oil, in hard margarine, ghee and cooking fat and as 'hidden' fats in cakes, biscuits, chocolate and puddings. They may be in the ingredients list as 'hydrogenated vegetable fat/oil'.

- **Unsaturated fats (or 'unsaturates')**. This group includes polyunsaturated fats and mono-unsaturated fats. In very small amounts these are essential to the body to provide certain vitamins and make foods more pleasant to eat. *These fats are still high in calories*. Unsaturated fats are found in vegetable oils, such as sunflower, corn, soya, rapeseed and olive oils, in soft margarine labelled 'high in polyunsaturates', in nuts and in oily fish such as sardines, herring mackerel, trout and pilchards.

Ways to substitute unsaturated fat for saturated fat

- Use a low fat poly/mono-unsaturated spread.
- Use a poly/mono-unsaturated fat in cooking.
- Try not to use *blended vegetable oil* (may be high in saturated fat).

Making a start

Making changes to your eating patterns usually means changing long-established habits related to shopping, cooking and eating. When you are planning such changes to your lifestyle, you can therefore help yourself to be more successful by thinking it through beforehand. This can help by drawing your attention to problems or difficulties that you may be able to prevent in advance.

How can you set yourself up so the changes you make are successful?

Below are some suggestions. Tick those that you think will be helpful to you. If you can think of any others, add them to the list.

- Stock your food cupboards with foods that do not trigger eating 'the wrong things'.
- Plan your shopping in advance so that you only buy suitable things.
- Carry suitable snacks with you.
- Plan eating times daily in advance.
- Have suitable snacks available in the car.

- Ask a friend, partner or work mate to encourage you.
- When cooking, avoid tasting as this may result in over-eating.
- Avoid unnecessary exposure to food.

What do you do when the going gets tough?

At times it can be quite difficult to maintain changes. It will take time for the changes you are making to become part of your everyday life. All those who try to change their behaviour occasionally find that they have done something that does not fit in with their plans. These one-off slip-ups, or lapses, often lead to feelings of guilt, which makes the individuals more susceptible to other slips and can eventually force them to abandon their changes altogether.

To help you to maintain new changes, or when things get difficult, it can help to think about what you can use to motivate yourself. Below are some suggestions:

- Talk to the friend or partner who agreed to encourage you.
- Remind yourself of the short-term and long-term benefits to your health.
- Review your achievements up until the present.
- Find healthy ways to treat yourself because of your achievements.

Changing your diet

- **Eat regular meals**. Try to plan your meals around starchy foods (such as bread, potatoes, rice, pasta and cereals) from day to day. This will help to keep your blood glucose in the normal range.
- **Try to cut down on fat**. Cut down on fried and fatty foods such as butter, margarine, cheese and fatty meats. These foods are high in calories and can make you gain weight. Choose reduced fat spreads and cheeses instead. Try skimmed or semi-skimmed milk.
- **Eat more high-fibre starchy carbohydrate foods**. The fibre in beans, peas, lentils and fruit is particularly good because it slows down the rate at which your body absorbs carbohydrate.
- **Aim to reduce your sugar intake**. Cut down on sugar, confectionery and sugary drinks. You can use artificial sweeteners such as saccharin, diet drinks and reduced sugar preserves.
- **Cut down on your salt intake**. Reduce salt added in cooking by using more herbs and spices instead. Gradually cut down on the salt you add to your food at the table.

- **Try to drink alcohol only in moderation**. People with diabetes should try to limit their intake of alcohol. Never drink on an empty stomach and always have something to eat with your drink, or shortly afterwards.
- **Avoid special diabetic foods**. They can be expensive and offer no special health benefit.

In changing your diet, it is important to set realistic goals that are actually achievable. There is nothing like success to increase motivation and enthusiasm. Look on changes as a positive opportunity to increase the enjoyment of eating and the variety of your diet – and appreciate any health aspects as an additional bonus.

Box 6. Key points about a healthy diet.

- Eat regularly.
- Include some starchy food with each meal, high-fibre versions if possible.
- Reduce your fat intake.
- Limit your sugar intake.
- Try to maintain you body weight and increase your physical activity.
- Use salt sparingly.
- Do not drink too much alcohol.

What about eating out and holidays?

“Of course, the fact that I have diabetes needs to be taken into account if I eat out or change jobs but it's not at the forefront of my mind. Anyway, you're always learning when you have diabetes.”

“At first, eating out and diabetes seemed like such a minefield. I thought 'what can I eat now that I have diabetes?' but I found that just making small changes to begin with really helps you.”

“I was a bit afraid to eat out with my friends at first, afraid I might embarrass them.”

Eating out

Increasingly, we have more and more meals away from home – eating in restaurants and pubs or grabbing sandwiches and takeaways on the run. However, food made away from home tends to be higher in fat and salt and lower in fibre than the home-made equivalent. As long as eating out is not the usual thing you do, then it should not be a problem, but if you eat out regularly look out for lower fat options, avoid items that are served in butter or cream, and are fried or battered. These are often loaded with fat because of the way they are prepared.

It is sometimes difficult to know what to do when eating out with friends who have made a special effort to prepare delicious food for you, which then turns out to be quite unsuitable. However, if you warn your friends in advance that you have diabetes and want to avoid food containing high concentrations of sugar, you will probably find it less embarrassing all round.

Holidays and travelling

If you are going abroad on holiday the same rules apply but obviously you may have to be extra careful if you do not understand the menu or are unfamiliar with some of the dishes. Some airlines offer 'special diabetic' meals on the plane. It is actually better to avoid them because they can be low in carbohydrate – caterers often do not realise that balance is the main thing, not cutting down on carbohydrate. Also it is a good idea to take extra carbohydrate in your hand luggage.

Parties and special events

With a little thought and pre-planning, you can feel free to go to any party and enjoy yourself as much as ever. The main considerations are that you will probably be eating later than usual, having different kinds of food and possibly dancing late into the night. When you are on insulin or on tablets, you will need to make certain adjustments to take account of these factors. You will need to eat more to allow for extra activities such as dancing. Dancing will mean that you have to have extra carbohydrate – the amount depending on how much energy you put into your performance!

HELPFUL TIPS! HELPFUL TIPS! HELPFUL TIPS! HELPFUL

There are various ways of 'handling' parties and special events:

- **Plan ahead**. Think about the event before you go. Try to anticipate the types of food you will face and the actions of other people. Think about your own desires to eat and the external pressures from others. Have a general idea of what you will eat. You can phone beforehand and ask what will be served. If you pre-plan your food intake, you will decrease the strength of your desire to eat what may not be best for you.

- **Eat before you go**. Do not go hungry to a party or special event. Everything will look good and you will forget that you only want to sample special foods. Have a salad or other low-calorie food before you go. (It is just like shopping for groceries: if you eat before you shop, you will not buy as much!) Furthermore, when you know you are going to be having a meal several hours later than normal, have a light snack before you go, then delay your injection until the food is ready.

- **Eat only special foods**. Stay away from the chips, crisps, dips, nuts and other foods that you can have any time. Use the chance to try new foods or foods you rarely have. Remember to make the best use of your calories.

- **Be the slowest eater**. Keep your eye on others and be the slowest eater at the event. Be the last to start and the last to finish. You will enjoy the food more and will feel satisfied with less. Pay attention to the texture, smell and subtleties of taste. This will stop the rapid and automatic eating that consumes so many calories.

- **Keep a proper perspective**. If you do eat more than you intend to, keep a positive attitude. Do not turn an event into more than it really is – just another day with meals and calories. In the scheme of a month or year's worth of eating, what can one day mean? One day's indiscretion should not ruin any eating plan. The trick is to bounce back. Your reaction to the eating is more important than the eating itself. Your attitudes are central to your ability to control your eating, both during and after the event.

Understanding and managing increasing physical activity

When a person who does not have diabetes takes exercise, the release of insulin from the pancreas is shut down, while other hormones are produced which cause the blood glucose level to rise. When you are taking insulin or sulphonylurea tablets, however, your insulin level continues to rise, and if you have had an injection into one of the limbs you are exercising, the insulin may be absorbed faster than usual.

Why is exercise important for people with diabetes?

Exercise is important for everyone. It helps us to look good and feel better about ourselves; it increases physical fitness; it reduces the risk of heart disease; it helps with weight control; and it improves muscle tone. Besides improving the body, exercise can also promote a positive, healthy outlook on life.

For people with diabetes, exercise offers even greater benefits. Most importantly, regular exercise can help to improve blood glucose control. Daily physical activity reduces the body's resistance to insulin and increases the body cells' sensitivity to insulin. Therefore, people with type 1 diabetes can keep tight control over their blood sugar levels with smaller amounts of insulin. The same applies to individuals with type 2 diabetes who need to take insulin or oral diabetes medications. Another benefit of exercise is that it can help to reduce blood fat levels, decreasing the risk of heart attack or stroke.

During moderate exercise, glucose stored in muscles is used up first. The muscles then begin using blood glucose, thus gradually lowering the blood glucose level. Even after exercising, the blood glucose continues to fall as the muscles replenish their glucose stores. It is also believed that some body cells respond better to insulin for up to several days after exercising. Since part of the problem in type 2 diabetes is inadequate insulin utilisation (inability of cells to respond to insulin), it is likely that regular exercise can help to keep body cells responsive to insulin continuously so that swings in blood glucose levels can be avoided.

How much exercise should you do?

In order for exercise to be effective, it usually must be practised vigorously for at least 15 minutes, three times a week. Daily exercise, of course, is better. However, consult with your diabetes team before starting any exercise programme so that you can develop one that will work best for you.

Why bother?

Many people avoid exercise because it is uncomfortable, takes time, or they feel embarrassed or unskilled. There are, however, great benefits from even small amounts of increased activity without the necessity for 'aerobics'. Physical activity and exercise are positive aspects of health – they generally involve doing something constructive. Activity is for everyone; our bodies are made to move and unless we keep moving the capacity for physical functioning becomes greatly reduced. Indeed many of the concerns associated with growing older are quite often more to do with inactivity.

It is not uncommon for people who are older or overweight to think that because they cannot run six miles or do an advanced level of aerobics, anything less is worthless, and they therefore do *no* physical activity. However, every bit of activity is important, even the odd few minutes can help to get you going. You can then build up by gradually extending the time you can sustain the activity, within your daily routine.

Still not convinced?

'It's too much like hard work. I'd never keep it up'

It will not seem to be hard work if you choose an activity you enjoy and build up slowly and gradually. As you get better you will enjoy it even more and you will not want to give it up.

'I haven't got time. My life is too busy'

Just 20 minutes two or three times a week can keep you feeling young and active. Once you start feeling the benefits, and your new activity becomes a habit, it will be much easier to fit into your routine.

'What I need is relaxation'

Exercise can be just the thing to help you to relax. It relieves stress by taking your mind off your problems. After a session of vigorous exercise, you will feel warm, comfortable and relaxed. You will notice the relaxing effect of some kinds of exercise even while you are doing them. Recent studies have shown that exercising can also help with depression, and you will probably find that it also helps you to sleep better.

'But doesn't it have to hurt to do you any good?'

No! If it hurts, then you are pushing yourself too hard. If you are in any pain, stop. If you feel uncomfortably out of breath, slow down or stop.

'It's too late for me – I'm past it!'

It is never too late. Anyone can get fitter. Whatever your age you can find a form of physical activity that will suit you. And the less fit you are to start with, the sooner you will notice the benefits.

'But isn't it bad for my heart?'

On the contrary, it helps to protect your heart. When you exercise, your muscles need more oxygen than usual, so your heart has to beat faster to pump more oxygen-carrying blood to them. Also, if you exercise regularly, your muscles get better at using oxygen and your heart pumps more blood with each beat, so it does not need to beat so quickly. As you get fitter you can exercise harder without overtaxing your heart. Regular exercise has other benefits too. It can help to control high blood pressure. It can also help to stop your arteries furring up, and over the years your risk of having a heart attack will be reduced.

'I'm not the sporty type'

Even if you did not like sport at school, there are now so many different activities, you are sure to be able to find one you enjoy. Just try different ones until you find the one that is right for you. Remember, walking is a very good form of exercise.

'I'd be too embarrassed'

Do not let embarrassment put you off increasing your physical activity – you would be missing out on too much! People of all shapes and sizes enjoy exercising and you will not feel uncomfortable or out of place if you choose an activity that is right for you.

'I couldn't bear all the sprains and strains'

You will only get these if you push yourself too hard, too soon. Or if you do an occasional session of hard exercise and nothing in between. If you start off gently and build up slowly, your risks of sprains and strains are very low. Exercise builds up strong muscles, which protect you from injury. When muscles are not used, for example when a broken leg is put in plaster, the muscles waste away and the leg gets thin and weak. But if muscles are used more than usual, for example for exercising, they get stronger and more efficient.

'If I can't do it properly, then what's the point of doing it at all?'

You do not have to go into serious training and get super fit or play competitive sports to gain benefits from exercise. Regular activity for just 20 or 30 minutes, two or three times a week, will go a long way towards helping you to stay in good shape.

'I'm too fat for that kind of thing'

Then you are just the type of person who will benefit most from some regular physical activity, especially if it is the stamina-building type. Exercising helps you to control your weight by burning up calories. If you burn up more calories than you eat, your body will start using up its own energy stores and fat will start to disappear. There is evidence that some people may still be burning up more calories than usual – sometimes for up to 24 hours – *after* they have finished exercising.

HELPFUL TIPS! HELPFUL TIPS! HELPFUL TIPS! HELPFUL

There are various ways of increasing your physical activity:

- **To get moving, increase activity in your day-to-day routine**. Increasing lifestyle activity is easy, takes little time, is not painful, does not require special clothes/equipment and helps you to feel better.

- **Use more effort than usual**. Find a more active way to do the things you usually do; for example, *lose the remote control for the television*, and get up and change the channels every time you want to watch another programme! Remember, *every bit of activity counts!*

- **Use the stairs instead of the lift**. Climbing stairs is a good way of keeping your leg muscles strong.

- **Walk more!** If you are not very active now, your first step to getting fitter is simply to walk more. When you walk, *walk faster*. Walking briskly for 20 to 30 minutes, two or three times a week, will soon build up your stamina. It is an ideal exercise.

- **Build up gradually**. It takes time to get fit. Work hard enough to make yourself a bit sweaty and out of breath, but not uncomfortably. That way there will also be less risk of sprains and strains.

- **Keep it up!** You cannot store fitness.

Are you struggling?

Sometimes becoming more active seems difficult to do because there are too many things stopping you and not enough things helping you.

- Identify the main things that are making it difficult to become more physically active:
  - Are they to do with yourself, for example, 'I haven't got the time?'
  - Are they to do with other people, for example, 'No one will come with me?'

- Are they to do with your surroundings, for example, 'There is nowhere suitable to walk?'
- Can you remove any of these or make them less important?
- Tackle the ones that seem easiest to deal with first.
- If you can release the brake a little, then you are more likely to be able to move forward.

Box 7.	Key points about physical activity.

- Being active helps you to feel good.
- It helps you to feel more energetic.
- It helps you to relax.
- It helps to improve your diabetes control.
- It helps to control your body weight.
- It improves your circulation and helps to protect against heart disease.
- It helps to prevent osteoporosis.

Understanding and managing the main goals of treatment

The main goal of any treatment programme is to bring glucose levels down to as close to normal as possible. By keeping blood sugar levels within the normal range, you can prevent short-term complications such as hypoglycaemia (low blood sugar) and hyperglycaemia (high blood sugar), and greatly reduce your risk of developing long-term complications, including kidney disease, cardiovascular disease, and nerve damage.

Understanding your role in treatment

You are the most important member of your treatment team because you are the one who lives with diabetes every day. It is up to you to monitor your blood glucose levels and to take any medications necessary to keep these levels within a normal range. It is up to you to make healthy food choices and to follow your physical activity programme. Ultimately, you are the person responsible for making important decisions about your care. Regardless of how many professionals are on your side, if you do not take steps to effectively manage your diabetes, you will be putting yourself at a greater risk of developing complications.

Monitoring your blood glucose levels

There are four essential components in all proper diabetes management treatment programmes:

- Monitoring your blood glucose levels.
- Following a healthy diet.
- Implementing and following a physical activity programme.
- Knowing how and when to take any medications that you are prescribed.

The point of all treatment for diabetes – whether it is diet, tablets or insulin – is to keep the levels of glucose in your bloodstream as close as possible to normal. The nearer you get to achieving this, the better you will feel, especially in the long term. There are two ways you can monitor glucose levels and your doctor or diabetes nurse will advise you about which one you should use and how often to do the checks. The two methods available are blood tests and urine tests, and neither is particularly difficult once you understand them.

The development of simple finger-prick blood-testing methods in the last few years has transformed life for patients taking insulin. Keeping a close check on your glucose levels is very useful when you are on insulin because it means that you can make adjustments to your dose depending on the results. When your diabetes is controlled by tablets and/or diet, urine tests can give you nearly as much information as blood tests and may be more convenient. There are also blood tests that can be performed in hospital, which measure an average blood glucose level over a period – which may be from two to eight weeks – before the test. We will now consider each of these approaches in turn.

Blood tests

There are two systems available for self-blood glucose monitoring (or SBMG as you may hear it called). Both give accurate results, and as well as helping you to improve your blood glucose control, they can be useful if you suspect you may be about to have a hypoglycaemic reaction. Taking an exact reading will either reassure you that all is well or confirm that you need to take action. Blood-testing strips are available on prescription but the special meters for reading them have to be purchased separately.

Urine tests

Glucose appears in your urine when your kidneys can no longer reabsorb the amount being filtered. The problem with urine testing is that this 'overflow point' is not the same for everyone. The correct term for this overflow point is the kidney (or renal) threshold. Some people who do not have diabetes have a low threshold, and they often need the glucose tolerance test described earlier to confirm the fact and explain why glucose has appeared in their urine.

The normal threshold is around a blood glucose level of 10 millimoles per litre (mmol/l), so for a person with diabetes, a negative urine test can mean that your blood glucose level is anywhere between 0 and 10 mmol/l, depending on your personal threshold. A positive test, on the other hand, does not tell you the exact level of blood glucose or by how much it exceeds your own personal threshold.

Despite this relative lack of accuracy, testing your urine and getting mostly negative results may be all you need to confirm that your diabetes is well under control, especially if you are being treated with diet and/or tablets.

What do the results tell you?

When you do either a blood test or a urine test, you are really measuring how effective your previous dose of insulin or tablet treatment has been. In other words, doing a test just before lunch will tell someone on insulin the effect of his or her early morning injection of short-acting insulin. In the same way, a pre-breakfast test will reflect the effectiveness of the previous night-time dose. The same interpretation applies in principle to tablets.

When the test result shows a high level of glucose, you may have to increase the size of your next dose of medication to restore the balance. This solves the problem in the short term, but ideally you want to prevent the problem arising in the first place by adjusting the dose that preceded the test. It is a good idea to vary the time of day when you do your test, and also to wait for a series of results over a period of, say, three to five days, before making too many adjustments. That way, you will see whether there is any pattern to the changes in your blood glucose level.

Until you have more experience of handling your diabetes, it would be better to consult your GP or someone in your diabetes care team before altering your insulin or tablet dosage. Later, when you have learned more about your body's reactions, you will be able to make the necessary adjustments on your own because you will know what works best for you.

Hospital monitoring

If you have type 1 diabetes, there may be situations where your medical advisers feel that it would be useful to assess the effectiveness of your treatment by means of more sophisticated blood tests. They are not a substitute for your own routine testing, but can give additional information that will help the doctor to decide whether your treatment needs adjustment. Both tests require a blood sample to be taken from a vein.

HbA1c – Glycated haemoglobin

This measures your average blood glucose level over a period of some six to eight weeks. Like all averages, however, it could be the result of lots of small variations or much larger swings in either direction. For this reason, it is not useful for making day-to-day adjustments of insulin treatment, but is a good guide as to whether your treatment is working well overall.

Box 8. **Key points about blood tests.**

- Blood tests provide more accurate information about glucose control.
- Blood tests are more helpful to exclude hypoglycaemia (low blood glucose).
- Urine tests are perfectly adequate for monitoring patients on diet control or low doses of the glucose-lowering tablets, but are not very helpful for alerting the patient to hypoglycaemia.

Following the treatment plan

It is very important that you follow the treatment that your doctor or diabetes nurse has advised. You will feel much better if you keep your blood glucose levels as near to normal as possible. You should aim for a level of 4–7 mmol/l before meals, rising to no higher that 10 mmol/l two hours after meals. Your diabetes team will advise you on what is best for you.

Summary

- Treatment for diabetes varies from person to person and will depend on your type of diabetes.

- Type 1 diabetes is treated by injections of insulin and a healthy diet, and regular exercise is recommended.

- Type 2 diabetes is treated by a healthy diet and exercise or by a combination of a healthy diet, exercise and tablets. Eventually people with type 2 diabetes may also need insulin injections.

- Whichever type of diabetes you have, your food choice helps to balance your blood glucose levels and your diet is therefore an essential part of your treatment.

- For people with diabetes, increasing daily physical activity levels can help to improve blood glucose control, reduce the body's resistance to insulin and increase the body cells' sensitivity to insulin.

- The main goal of any treatment programme is to bring glucose levels down to as close to normal as possible.

- You are the most important member of your treatment team because you are the one who lives with diabetes every day. It is your responsibility to monitor your blood glucose levels, to take any medications necessary to keep these levels within a normal range, to make healthy food choices and to follow your physical activity programme.

- It is very important that you follow the treatment that your doctor or diabetes care team has advised.

Understanding and managing lifestyle change

6

While medication is key in helping to control blood glucose levels, it is only one aspect of treating your diabetes. Diabetes is a condition in which you can largely help yourself and this inevitably involves making some changes to your lifestyle.

> **"**A strict diet that a dietician or a doctor gives me, I keep to it for about three weeks. I lose weight, but I feel really awful and can't keep on with it and then I just have to stop it.**"**

> **"**Obviously, if you're that bad you should do the things they tell you, but as long as I remain more or less as I am, it'll not bother me. I'll just carry on as I am.**"**

> **"**I did join the gym at one point but I gave up on that because I wasn't going, there always seemed to be a reason why I couldn't go, and so it was just a waste of money.**"**

We now know that many of the risk factors for the major illnesses in society today are due in part to our own behaviour and how we live our lives, for example smoking and overeating. This recognition that our own behaviour is a key component in both the cause and prevention of disease has led to numerous efforts to change unhealthy behaviours and lifestyles. However, lifestyle change is often the most difficult and challenging aspect of care for both patients and health-care professionals.

Research has therefore focused on individuals' beliefs and feelings about health and illness from a variety of different perspectives, which provide a basis for understanding what determines our behaviour and how we might change it, and highlights important targets on which we can focus to help to change individuals lifestyles. This chapter will focus on managing lifestyle change and discuss motivation for change, it provides a psychological model of how changes occur and discusses the strategies that can be used to help to promote and maintain successful lifestyle change.

Motivation for change

It seems clear that a person's motivation for change is affected by a variety of conditions, some of which are external to the individual and some of which are internal. Psychologists suggest that motivation should not be thought of as a characteristic that an individual either has or has not – a kind of personality problem. Rather, motivation can best be seen as a *state* of readiness or *eagerness* to change, which may fluctuate from one time or situation to another. Importantly, from this perspective, we can see that this *state* is therefore one that can be influenced.

One helpful model of how change occurs has been developed by psychologists who have sought to understand how and why people change, either on their own or with the help of health care professionals. They have described a series of stages through which people pass in the course of changing a problem, and this has been portrayed as a 'wheel of change' (see Figure 3). Within this approach, motivation can be understood as a person's present state or stage of readiness for change. This state or stage of readiness is an internal state that is influenced by external factors.

This 'wheel of change' can be drawn with five stages; the fact that it is a wheel, a circle, reflects the reality that in almost any change process, it is normal for most of us to go around the process several times before finally achieving stable change, and it recognises that relapse is a normal occurrence for most of us when changing behaviours. Also, by discriminating between different stages of readiness for change, this model implies that, depending upon where you are in the process of change, different skills, information and strategies for change may be needed.

Stage 1: Not interested in change

In this first stage people are not aware of the fact that they have a problem and therefore they do not think seriously about change. Others may recognise

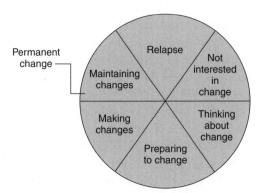

Figure 3. Stages of change model. Adapted from Prochaska, J.O. and DiClemente, C.C.D. (1982) Transtheoretical therapy: Toward a more integrative model of change. *Psychotherapy: Theory, Research and Practice, 19,* 176–288

that there is a problem and that change is necessary, but it does not relate to their behaviour. During this stage there is usually a lack of personal knowledge of the problem. The awareness of having problems often brings along a loss of self-esteem and confidence and people are likely to defend themselves against the idea of having problems. People tend to have certain built-in defence mechanisms against a decrease in self-esteem and confidence. This defence is sticking to your own opinion. If a person at this stage would want to change anything, this would probably not be that person's own behaviour but the behaviour of others – for example, a nagging friend, family member or health-care professional. So, an individual at this stage does not really need to be told what to do but rather should be given more information and feedback to raise his or her awareness of the problem and the possibility of change.

Stage 2: Thinking about change

In this stage we realise that there are problems and start thinking about possible ways to get rid of or control the problem, but the definite decision to change has not yet been reached. The main worry at this stage is the fear of losing something pleasant, that we actually enjoy doing – like smoking, for example – and the fear of whether we will manage to solve the problem adequately. During this stage, our thinking is really like an old-fashioned two-sided balance weighing scale, and we are usually ambivalent about changing. On the one side there are arguments for changing what we do but on the other side there are arguments against. What we need at this stage is something to help to tip the balance in favour of change.

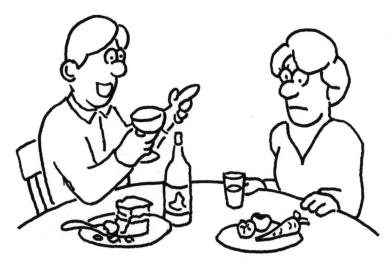

Eating differently can be hard

Stage 3: Preparing to change

This is in fact not really a separate stage but is seen as the transitional stage from thinking about change to actively making changes and is characterised by a decision making process. At this stage, we weigh up all the pros and cons connected to the present situation and decide whether we are going to make changes or not. Help in developing an individual action plan (Box 9) and finding a change strategy that is acceptable to you, appropriate for you and effective can be very important at this stage.

Box 9. **Making an action 'plan'.**

The essential elements of an 'action plan' are:

- What specifically are you going to do?
- Where and when?
- For long?
- Who with?
- What is the goal?
- How will you reward yourself when you have achieved it?
- What will you do if you 'slip' from your plan?
- What are the potential barriers to you doing this?
- How will you overcome them?

Stage 4: Making changes

In this stage, people engage in particular actions intended to bring about a change, and first successes give us a new feeling of confidence and help us to lose our fear of not being able to make any alterations in our behaviour. Usually, people around us notice these changes and make some comments! Although people often progress through this stage very rapidly, it is also the stage in which improvement is most visible, and individuals try to stabilise the changes that they have so far made to prevent a relapse into the old unwanted behaviour.

Stage 5: Maintaining changes

Making a change, however, does not guarantee that the change will be maintained. Obviously, human experience is filled with good intentions and initial changes, followed by minor ('slips') or major ('relapses') steps backward. During this stage the challenge is to sustain the change that you have accomplished and to prevent relapse, and this will require a different set of skills and strategies than those needed to accomplish the change in the first place.

Relapse

Finally, if 'relapse' occurs, the task is to start around the wheel again rather than getting stuck in this stage. Slips and relapses are normal and expected occurrences as a person tries to change any long-standing pattern. The diabetes team is there to help you to avoid discouragement and demoralisation, to continue thinking about changing your lifestyle, to renew your determination, to resume making efforts to change, and to maintain the changes.

Box 10.	Key questions to ask yourself about readiness to change.	
Importance (Why?)	*Confidence* (How? What?)	*Readiness* (When?)
Is it worth while? Why should I?	Can I? How will I do it?	Should I do it now? What about other priorities?
How will I benefit?	How will I cope with x, y or z?	
What will change? At what cost to me or my family? Do I really want to? Will it make a difference?	Will I succeed if......? What change?	

What strategies can you use to help you change your lifestyle?

Several specific strategies have consistently been found to be useful in changing lifestyle, that lead to big improvements in health for individuals with diabetes.

Self-monitoring

Self-monitoring involves the systematic observation and recording of target behaviours, including the use of food and activity diaries to record calorie intake, fat grams, food groups, conditions or situations when overeating is common, and frequency, duration and/or intensity of exercise. While you may not always be accurate in the reporting of dietary and exercise behaviours, the primary purpose of self-monitoring is to increase your awareness of any problematic dietary and activity patterns and the factors that influence how you behave. Self-monitoring is associated consistently with improved treatment outcomes, and most people report that it is one of the most helpful self-management tools.

Stimulus control

Much of our behaviour is habitual and automatic; triggers or cues exist to initiate routine behaviours and, in this way, a person does not consciously have to think about what to do next. Stimulus control involves identifying these environmental triggers or cues that are associated for you with, for example, overeating and underactivity. Modifying these cues, and therefore changing the environment around you, may increase your success in sustaining your behaviour changes. Controlling cues associated with overeating or inactivity can facilitate long-term maintenance because exposure to these cues may precipitate relapse. There are numerous ways to implement this strategy, depending on the individual. Prompting people to exercise through weekly telephone calls, for example, has been found to significantly enhance adherence to a walking programme. In addition, eliminating the availability of snack foods in the house or restricting eating to particular rooms can be helpful.

Cognitive behaviour therapy (CBT) interventions

This strategy involves getting people to address their thoughts and beliefs about themselves and their problems and teaching them to actively challenge and change aspects of their internal dialogue. This is particularly important because, for example, some individuals hold unrealistic beliefs about how much weight they can lose through a treatment programme and the benefits that weight loss will have on their lives. Researchers have found, for example, that people in weight management studies had weight loss expectations that were substantially different from what was realistically achievable. While many people lose about 10 per cent of their initial weight during treatment, thus reducing their risks for developing further complications of diabetes, this moderate amount of weight loss was much less than the weight loss that these individuals defined as an acceptable outcome.

Stress management

Stress is a primary predictor of relapse and overeating, and stress management training is an important part of most programmes. Stress management involves teaching people with diabetes methods for reducing stress and tension, including diaphragmatic breathing, muscle relaxation or meditation (see page 47 above). In addition, stress inoculation involves having people visualise stressful situations while practising their relaxation skills, therefore allowing them to practise managing stressors in a safe environment and improving their confidence in coping with stressful situations. These techniques are designed to reduce tension and associated changes that occur in your body in response to stressors and have been found to be very effective for numerous health-related problems, including diabetes.

Relapse prevention

It is important to be prepared for lapses in following your treatment plan. Lapses are a normal part of any health behaviour change plan and you need to recognise and anticipate situations that might cause a lapse. For example, many studies have found that negative emotions and social situations, such as holidays or parties, are associated with lapses. Your diabetes team can help you to develop coping strategies to manage lapses and prevent full relapses.

Social support

Social support is an important component of successful diabetes management. Many studies have found that individuals with higher levels of social support tend to do better, for example, in weight management programmes or keeping to their diabetes treatments. Social support may involve your family in the treatment programme, you may be required to participate in a community-based programme, or be involved in some outside social activity. Friends and family support may be particularly useful because it helps people to learn greater self-acceptance, develop new norms for interpersonal relationships and manage stressful work or family-related situations.

Barriers to change

It is important to identify perceived barriers to change. Individuals with diabetes frequently have a higher rate of other medical conditions, which may substantially increase their discomfort during physical activity for example and limit their endurance and flexibility. Researchers have found that a group of significantly overweight women who were tested during walking and cycling exercises walked more slowly and had more breathing difficulties than normal weight individuals. In addition, they reported high degrees of perceived exertion and pain. These results suggest that walking, which is generally considered to be a moderate-intensity activity, may actually be more intense for very overweight individuals due to the greater relative oxygen cost of walking associated with increased body size.

Overweight diabetic people, therefore, may be more likely to perceive even moderate-intensity activity, such as walking, as exerting and painful which may have a negative impact on actually doing it. Thus the presence or one or more other medical conditions may present a significant barrier to starting or maintaining a physical activity programme. Other barriers include those that affect any individual, such as lack of time, equipment, facilities, childcare or family support.

Similarly, other important barriers to lifestyle change in the overweight diabetic person may be programme-based shortcomings. For example, the foundation of many physical activity programmes is based on research that has focused on benefits to the heart and lungs. This can have the unfortunate side-effect of discouraging individuals from starting activity programmes because they may mistakenly assume that small amounts of low-intensity activity, which is where most overweight diabetic individuals will begin, have little health value. Importantly, however, low- to moderate-intensity physical activity programmes for diabetic people initially may be very helpful in improving psychological well-being, functional status and adherence, paving the way for participation in more intense programmes.

Strategies to promote adherence

There are several basic strategies that can be utilised to help you to keep to your treatment regimens and lifestyle changes.

First, developing good rapport with your diabetes care team is very important. This can involve discussing barriers to treatment and attending education sessions about the need for intervention and reviewing the expected course and outcomes. Education of the individual with diabetes is an important part of most treatment programmes and works to address many of the barriers related to either the individual or the health-care professional. Examples include ensuring that you understand the dietary and activity prescriptions by writing them down, discussing your beliefs about your diabetes and how diet and physical activity may benefit you, providing clear information about any complications and related conditions and how lifestyle change may be helpful in improving these conditions, and assessing your expectations. Building alliances with the diabetes team is a very important aspect of improving treatment adherence and addressing important psychological and social barriers to dietary change and physical activity for people with diabetes.

Second, treatment programmes can be modified so that they are more easily incorporated into your lifestyle. For example, the emphasis on moderate lifestyle physical activities is one way to make physical activity initially more accessible to overweight individuals. It can be helpful to include people in the development of management goals and encourage them to increase their activity intensity and duration gradually. Giving feedback about progress and providing a way for individuals to monitor progress through self-monitoring is one of the most effective methods for enhancing activity and dietary adherence and promoting weight loss. Furthermore, the beneficial effect of social support has been demonstrated for physical activity, dietary change and weight management.

Summary

- Lifestyle change is often the most challenging and difficult aspect of care.

- Motivation for change is affected by a variety of conditions, some of which are external to the individual and some of which are internal.

- One helpful model of how change occurs describes a series of stages through which people pass in the course of changing a problem. Depending on where you are in the process of change, different skills, information and strategies for change may be needed.

- In changing lifestyle, several specific strategies that lead to big improvements in health for individuals with diabetes have consistently been found to be useful.

Living with diabetes

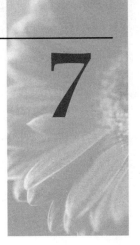

As you learn to live with diabetes you will gradually
realise that you can lead a normal life, and
provided that you understand the condition you
can probably do almost anything you wish!

> **"**The thing about living with diabetes is it makes you focus on yourself all
> the time, you need to think about where you are and what you are doing in
> terms of food, medicines, etc. – it can make you very self-orientated. **"**

> **"**Coming to terms with living with diabetes takes time, and no one can
> tell you how long it will be before you overcome all those initial feelings of
> anger, guilt, 'why me'. **"**

It would be impossible to focus on every aspect of daily living with diabetes. Instead,
this chapter will discuss a broad range of issues from taking part in sports, issues
related to work, managing other illnesses, driving, alcohol and smoking.

Diabetes and sports

People with diabetes have reached the top in many sports and the vast majority
of sports are perfectly safe for people with diabetes. The problem lies in those
sports where loss of control due to a hypo (i.e. hypoglycaemic reaction) could be
dangerous, not only to you but also to your fellow participants or to spectators.
Swimming is an example of a potentially dangerous sport but by taking certain
precautions, such as never swimming alone and keeping your glucose tablets on
the side of the pool, it is safe to swim. However, in other sports, for example motor
racing, the risks of serious injury in the case of a hypo are even greater. For
this reason the governing bodies of these high-risk sports discourage people with
diabetes from taking part. Discouragement does not necessarily mean a total ban;
the restrictions may vary depending on whether your treatment is diet, diet and

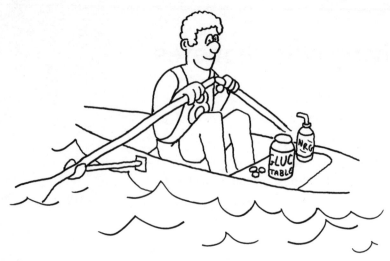

Sport is healthy, you just need to be prepared

tablets, or insulin. You can always contact the governing bodies of the particular sport that interests you and find out what, if any, restrictions they impose.

Diabetes and work

It is especially important to tell people at work about your diabetes, particularly if you are on insulin or the type of tablets that might make you have a hypo. Most people combine work with diabetes without any problems but shift work or working irregular hours may need a little extra adjustment with your medications as most insulin regimens, for example, are designed around a 24-hour clock. Shift workers usually complain that they are just settling into one routine when everything changes and they have to start again. It is difficult to generalise about shift work or irregular working hours as there are so many different patterns, but you should get help with this from your diabetes team, and employers are generally much more sympathetic if they know that you are doing your best to remedy the problem.

You should definitely warn fellow employees that you might be subject to a hypo. Tell your workmates that if they find you acting in a peculiar way they must get you to take some sugar. Warn them also that you may not be very cooperative at the time and may even resist their attempts to help you. Some people find it difficult to admit to their colleagues that they have diabetes but, if you keep it a secret, you run the risk of causing a scare by having a bad hypo and being taken to hospital by ambulance for treatment. This kind of situation is best avoided.

Ignorance and fear are the two main obstacles facing people with diabetes when looking for jobs and dealing with employers. You can be helped by the

Disability Discrimination Act 1995 (DDA). This makes it illegal for most employers to treat people with disabilities differently from other employees. Although most people with diabetes do not consider themselves disabled, diabetes is covered under the Act, because of other people's prejudices. If you need advice about getting a job or dealing with a particular situation in your present employment, the diabetes team at your clinic should be able to provide you with the relevant information and the Careline at Diabetes UK can give you more general supporting information.

Diabetes and other illnesses

Everybody gets colds and 'flu from time to time, and these, like other illnesses, can affect the control of your diabetes. The most likely result is that your blood glucose level will rise, so you need to make frequent checks to test whether this is happening, especially if you are on insulin. Because any illness can be potentially dangerous for people with diabetes, it is essential that you speak with your doctor and get specific instructions about self-care during sick days. You will need to know how often you should monitor your blood glucose when you are sick, when you will need to take more or less of your insulin or diabetes medication, and which over-the-counter medications are safe for you to use. By getting all the important information before you get sick, you will be prepared to take good care of yourself when, and if, it happens.

Type 1 diabetes

Many people think that if they are not eating they should not take their insulin, otherwise they will have a hypo. In fact, the opposite is the case. Your blood glucose level is much more likely to be too high than too low in these circumstances. Even if you have a stomach bug such as gastro-enteritis and are being sick constantly, you will still need some insulin to keep your glucose under control. If you cannot keep any fluids down, you must call your doctor immediately. You may have to go into hospital until you are again able to eat and drink.

Type 2 diabetes

Continuing to take your tablets when you are not able to eat or drink may cause a hypoglycaemic reaction. You may need a lower dose while you are ill, but unless you are monitoring your blood glucose regularly, you may need your doctor's advice on how to make the adjustment. If your illness does not settle down quickly, you may be admitted to hospital for a few days.

> **HELPFUL TIPS! HELPFUL TIPS! HELPFUL TIPS! HELPFUL**
>
> There are various ways to manage your diabetes when you are ill:
>
> - Don't stop your insulin or tablets.
> - Test your blood glucose level and urine frequently.
> - Drink plenty of unsweetened fluids.
> - Try to eat regularly – soup, milky drinks, Complan are useful alternatives to solid food.
> - Know when and where to contact your diabetes care team.

Diabetes and driving

Anyone whose diabetes is treated by diet alone does not require to inform the DVLA (Driving and Vehicle Licensing Agency). If your diabetes is treated by tablets or insulin, then you must declare this when applying for a driving licence. If you already hold a driving licence, then you must declare your diabetes to the DVLA as soon as you have been diagnosed. When you have notified the DVLA, they will send you a form asking for details about your diabetes and the names of any doctors you see regularly. They will also ask you to sign a declaration allowing your doctors to disclose medical details about your condition. There is usually no difficulty over someone with diabetes obtaining a licence to drive.

If you are treated with tablets, you will be able to obtain an unrestricted licence, providing you undertake to inform the DVLA of any change in your treatment or if you develop any complications of diabetes. If you are treated by insulin, the licence will be valid for only three years instead of up to the age of 70, which is applicable to most people in the UK. It is the risk of sudden and severe hypoglycaemia that makes people liable to this form of discrimination. In general the only people who have difficulty in obtaining a licence are those on insulin with very erratic control and a history of hypos causing unconsciousness. Once their condition has been controlled and severe hypos have been abolished, they can reapply for a licence with confidence. If you are renewing your licence, you may not be able to drive a minibus or a small lorry over 3–5 tonnes, as legislation has recently changed. For more information contact Diabetes UK.

Motor insurance is another problem for the driver with diabetes. Failure to inform your insurance company of your diabetes may make your cover invalid, in which case the consequences could be very serious. The insurance company usually asks your doctor to complete a form. Unfortunately there may be financial penalties for having diabetes and some insurance companies will load your premium. Again, contact Diabetes UK about this because they have set up a number of services, including home and motor insurance services, seeking to provide a better deal for people with diabetes.

HELPFUL TIPS! HELPFUL TIPS! HELPFUL TIPS! HELPFUL

There are various ways in which you can have diabetes and be a safe driver:

- Always carry food/glucose in your car.
- If you feel at all hypo, stop your car, take some glucose and move into the passenger seat.
- Check that your blood glucose level is above 5 mmol/l before driving off again.
- On a long journey, check your blood glucose level every few hours.

Diabetes and alcohol

Most people with diabetes drink alcohol and it is perfectly safe to do so. However, it is important to be aware that if you are treated with insulin, alcohol makes the occurrence of a hypo more likely and this increased risk continues for some time after you stop drinking. When someone has a hypo a number of hormones are produced that make the liver release glucose into the bloodstream. If that person has drunk some alcohol, even as little as two pints of beer or a double measure of spirits, the liver will not be able to release glucose and hypo reactions will be more sudden and more severe. This effect may be compounded by the fact that alcohol alters your perception and you may be less aware of your hypo symptoms. Therefore, when you are under the influence of alcohol you are not in the best shape to react appropriately and quickly.

Most alcoholic drinks also contain some carbohydrate, which tends to increase the glucose in the blood. The overall effect therefore of a particular alcoholic drink depends on the proportions of alcohol to carbohydrate. However, alcohol is high in calories, so if you are trying to lose weight you will need to cut down on your alcohol intake.

Always have something to eat with or shortly after your drink, maybe a sandwich or snack or something starchy like crisps. Remember, a hypo can happen several hours after you have finished drinking, so have an extra starchy snack afterwards. It is also worth taking a blood test before you go to sleep.

Diabetes and smoking

One of the most positive things you can do if you have diabetes is **stop smoking!** Smoking is a danger not only to the lungs because it causes cancer, but it also leads to hardening of the arteries, affecting chiefly the heart, brain and legs. Having diabetes means that you already run a higher than usual risk of damaged blood vessels, which can lead to certain conditions including heart attacks, kidney damage, strokes and problems with the blood supply to your legs. The risks for people with diabetes who smoke are therefore multiplied.

The benefits of giving up smoking are immediate. Only 20 minutes after you quit, your blood pressure and pulse rate return to normal. After 24 hours, carbon monoxide has left your body and the lungs start to clear themselves. Traces of nicotine begin to vanish within 48 hours of your last cigarette. You will soon notice a greatly improved sense of taste and smell and should feel more energetic. Breathing will become easier and your circulation will improve, making walking and running a lot easier. In the long term you are reducing your risk of serious conditions that pose a greater than average threat for people with diabetes, such as heart disease, kidney and eye problems.

A lot of support is now available for people who want to give up smoking, and your diabetes care team should be able to give you advice on whom to contact. You can also call Quitline on 0800 002200 for support and information, including details of local stop smoking support groups and information on various methods, including nicotine patches and chewing gum.

Summary

- As you learn to live with diabetes you will gradually realise that you can lead a normal life, and provided that you understand the condition you can probably do almost anything you wish!

- People with diabetes have reached the top in many sports and the vast majority of sports are perfectly safe for people with diabetes.

- It is especially important to tell people at work about your diabetes, particularly if you are on insulin or the type of tablets that might make you have a hypo.

- Another illness such as a cold or the 'flu can be potentially dangerous for people with diabetes, so it is essential that you speak with your doctor or diabetes care team and get specific instructions about self-care during those times when you have another illness.

- Anyone whose diabetes is treated by diet alone does not need to inform the DVLA (Driving and Vehicle Licensing Agency). If your diabetes is treated by tablets or insulin, then you must declare this when applying for a driving licence.

- Most people with diabetes drink alcohol and it is perfectly safe for them to do so. However, it is important to be aware that if you are treated with insulin, alcohol makes having a hypo more likely to occur and this increased risk continues for some time after you stop drinking.

- One of the most positive things you can do if you have diabetes is to give up smoking! Smoking is a danger not only to the lungs because it causes cancer, but because it leads to hardening of the arteries, affecting chiefly the heart, brain and legs.

Where can I get help?

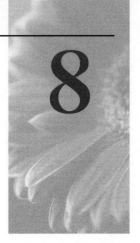

8

The limitations of the traditional diabetes clinic have encouraged the establishment of district diabetes centres, and expert advice and help is available throughout the week, not just in clinic hours, for anyone with diabetes.

> 66 Coming to terms with all the confused feelings as well as all the other practical things involved in living with diabetes can be very daunting, you definitely need to know where you can get some help to deal with it all. 99

> 66 It is a comfort to know that there are people out there who are trained and understand what is happening to you. 99

> 66 One of the worst things at the beginning is that you have to meet so many different health people, the doctor and nurse and dietician and that, it's all a bit mind boggling. 99

Now that you have been diagnosed with diabetes you will be visiting your GP and clinic not only when you have a problem with your diabetes but also when you are feeling perfectly well and for your routine diabetes reviews. You will be meeting a number of different health care professionals and will come to realise that diabetes care takes place at a number of different levels in the NHS. It is important for you to be aware of all these different professionals and levels so that you can make sure that you receive the best possible standards of care. This chapter, therefore, aims to describe (a) the types of care you can expect from the NHS, both at diagnosis and on an ongoing basis, (b) who the members of the diabetes care team are and their differing roles and responsibilities in looking after you and, (3) most importantly, your own role in managing your diabetes.

Diabetes clinics

The long-term care required by people with diabetes is organised in different ways from district to district. Traditional means of providing care are based upon attendance at a hospital diabetes clinic. Increasingly, however, the concept of 'shared care' – that is, care shared between the hospital and the general practice team – is being employed, and GPs are paid a fee for providing a programme of care, often in the form of a 'mini-clinic', approved by the local Family Health Services Authority. With this system many people with diabetes can be cared for principally by the primary health care team. Certain groups, such as children, adolescents or pregnant women with diabetes and those with specific complications or difficulties in management, will often require the specialised care of the hospital clinic or diabetes centre.

Though often based in or near the district general hospital, the diabetes centres are devoted to the provision of diabetes care throughout the district, and are a major and greatly valued resource for primary health care teams, patients and careers. These centres act as a focus for local organisation of diabetes services and coordination with general practitioners, and as centres for educational resources and programmes for people with diabetes, their carers and health-care professionals. With specialist facilities and experienced staff dedicated to diabetes care, the centre environment appears more conducive to treatment, teaching and learning.

The diabetes care team

Whether an individual with diabetes is cared for principally by a general practice team or by a hospital diabetes specialist team, it is now widely recognised that care is best provided by groups of health-care professionals with their own particular skills, working closely together. The teams include a consultant physician, diabetes specialist nurse, dietitian, chiropodist, general practitioner and practice nurse. They can also call upon the skills of a psychologist, ophthalmologist, nephrologist, neurologist, vascular and orthopaedic surgeons, obstetricians, midwifes and other specialists as necessary.

The **consultant physician** responsible for diabetes services has a special interest in diabetes. Such specialists are often referred to as diabetologists. In some districts, however, a general physician runs the clinic. One paediatrician in each district should have a specialist interest and knowledge of diabetes in children, and be part of a named and experienced paediatric diabetes team.

One of the most important innovations in diabetes care over recent years has been the increasing involvement of **diabetes specialist nurses** in providing care. Their main function involves educating, advising and counselling people with diabetes about all aspects of living with diabetes. They can play a pivotal role in coordinating the care provided by the entire team. They are usually based at the diabetes centre or hospital clinic, but will also liaise with general practices, and visit people in their own homes.

The **dietitians** are also essential members of the diabetes team. They assess eating patterns and advise on all aspects of healthy eating. **Chiropodists** also play an essential role in preventing the development of foot problems by providing education on foot care, and by assessing and treating as early as possible any foot problems that arise.

The **general practitioner** has overall responsibility for routine clinical care. He or she ensures that each person with diabetes receives effective surveillance of eyes, kidneys, feet and cardiovascular status in order that modifiable risk factors are picked up and treated early. The GP may have responsibility for identification and management of diabetic complications, and for identifying those individuals who require specialist hospital services. The **practice nurse** is responsible for providing education and advice, and coordinating care with other members of the team. He or she can also provide local social and psychological support for people with diabetes and their families.

Education of the individual with diabetes is an integral part of diabetes care. Each individual is responsible for how his or her diabetes is controlled, so the more that the person understands the condition itself and how to treat it, the more effective will the treatment be. All members of the professional team play a role in education, and teaching may take place either on a one-to-one basis, in group sessions, or both. Every contact between the person with diabetes and the health professional should be regarded as an opportunity for the education of both.

When diabetes is first diagnosed, support from the professional team is essential. Instruction about the condition and its treatment, advice about adapting lifestyle, and counselling about the implications are all vital. Continuing education, ready access to any member of the team when necessary, and a full formal annual medical review to assess, control and check for the development of complications should always be available.

Diabetes UK

Diabetes UK, the new name of the British Diabetic Association, is the leading charity working for people with diabetes. It is dedicated to helping people with diabetes, their carers, families and friends. The main aim of this organisation is to improve the lives of people with diabetes and to work towards a future without diabetes. Diabetes UK has produced a booklet setting out the standards of care you should expect from the National Health Service (NHS) and your role in managing your own diabetes, which includes the following:

1   What you should expect from the NHS

You should receive all health services without discrimination because of age, lifestyle, gender, ethnicity, class, religion, disability, sexuality or your ability to pay. There are several new initiatives, which aim to make best practice the norm wherever you receive your care. The initiatives have also been set up to reduce the medical complications associated with diabetes. In England and Wales there are new standards for diabetes (National Service Framework for Diabetes) and in Scotland there is the Scottish Diabetes Framework. These frameworks set out standards of care that will be implemented over the next few years in order to bring about improvements to diabetes care throughout the UK.

2 What care you should expect from your diabetes care team

To achieve the best possible diabetes care, you need to work together with health-care professionals as equal members of the diabetes care team. It is essential that you understand your diabetes as well as possible so that you are an effective member of this team.

When you have just been diagnosed, your diabetes care team should:

- Give you a full medical examination.
- Work with you to agree a care plan which suits you and includes diabetes management goals. This may take the form of a personal record for you to keep.
- Arrange for you to talk with a diabetes specialist nurse or practice nurse who will explain what diabetes is and discuss your individual treatment and the equipment you will need to use.
- Arrange for you to talk with a dietitian who will assess your current eating habits and advise on how to fit your usual diet in with your diabetes.
- Tell you about your diabetes and the beneficial effects of a healthy diet, exercise and good diabetes control.
- Discuss the effects of diabetes on your job, driving, insurance, prescription charges and, if you are a driver, whether you need to inform the DVLA or your insurance company.
- Provide you with regular and appropriate information and education.
- Give you information about your local voluntary diabetes groups.

Once your diabetes is reasonably controlled, you should:

- Have access to your diabetes care team at least once a year. In this session, it is important to take the opportunity to discuss how your diabetes affects *you* as well as your diabetes control.

- Be able to contact any member of your diabetes care team for specialist support and advice, in person or by phone.
- Have further education sessions when you are ready for them.
- Have a formal medical annual review once a year with a doctor experienced in diabetes.

On a regular basis, your diabetes care team should:

- Provide continuity of care, ideally from the same doctors and nurses.
- Work with you to continually review your care plan, including your diabetes management through regular reviews.
- Encourage you to share in decisions about your treatment or care.
- Encourage you to manage your own diabetes in hospital after discussion with your doctor, if you are well enough to do so and that is what you wish to happen.
- Organise pre- and post-pregnancy advice, together with an obstetric hospital team, if you are planning to become or are already pregnant.
- Encourage a carer to visit with you, to keep that person up to date on diabetes so that he or she can make informed judgements about diabetes care.
- Provide you with educational sessions and appointments if you wish.
- Give you advice on the effects of diabetes and its treatments when you are ill or taking other medication.

3 Your responsibilities

Effective diabetes care is normally achieved by teamwork, between you and your diabetes care team. Looking after your diabetes and changing your lifestyle to fit in with the demands of diabetes is hard work and you will not always get it right, none of us does, but your diabetes care team is there to support you. Ask questions and request more information, especially if you are uncertain or worried about your diabetes and/or treatment. Remember, the most important person in the team is you.

4 Annual review

It is important to remember that your annual review is to enable you to lead a normal and healthy life. It must be about what you want and need as well as what health-care professionals recommend. It should usually include laboratory tests and investigations, physical examinations, and time to discuss lifestyle issues and current problems or barriers to good diabetes self-management.

Summary

- It is important for you to be aware of all the different health care professionals and different levels in the NHS involved in your diabetes care so that you can make sure that you receive the best possible standards of care.

- Traditional means of providing care are based upon attendance at a hospital diabetes clinic. Increasingly, many people with diabetes can be cared for principally by the GP and primary health care team.

- It is now widely recognised that care is best provided by groups of health-care professionals, with their own particular skills, working closely together.

- The diabetes care team includes a consultant physician, diabetes specialist nurse, dietitian, chiropodist, general practitioner and practice nurse. They can also call upon the skills of a psychologist, ophthalmologist, nephrologist, neurologist, vascular and orthopaedic surgeons, obstetricians, midwifes and other specialists as necessary.

- Diabetes UK, the leading charity working for people with diabetes, has produced a booklet setting out the standards of care you should expect from the National Health Service (NHS) and your role in managing your diabetes.

- Your annual review is to enable you to lead as normal and as healthy a life as possible. It should usually include laboratory tests and investigations, physical examinations and time to discuss lifestyle issues and current problems or barriers to good diabetes self-management.

Where can I get more information?

National Service Frameworks (NSF) England

For copies of the *National Service Framework for Diabetes: Standards and Delivery Strategy for England*, contact:

Department of Health
PO Box 777, London SE1 6XH

or log on to:

www.doh.gov.uk/nsf/diabetes

NSF patient information *Living with Diabetes – Your Future Health and Wellbeing* is downloadable from the Diabetes UK website:

www.diabetes.org.uk/infocentre/response/nsf.pdf

or is available from the Department of Health (see above).

Diabetes UK

1. Diabetes UK, which is the new name for the British Diabetic Association, is an independent registered charity, dedicated to caring for people with diabetes in a number of ways, including care services, research, publications, promoting public awareness and links to professional organisations.

2. For information on joining Diabetes UK, educational events for all people with diabetes, or Diabetes UK local voluntary groups throughout the UK contact:

Diabetes UK
10 Parkway, London NW1 7AA
Telephone: 020 7424 1000
Email: info@diabetes.org.uk
Website: www.diabetes.org.uk

3. Diabetes UK Careline offers information and support on all aspects of diabetes. Trained staff provide a confidential service taking general enquiries on diabetes from people with diabetes, their careers and from health-care professionals.

For further information contact:

Diabetes UK Careline
10 Parkway, London NW1 7AA

Telephone: 020 7424 1030 (operates a translation service)
Email: careline@diabetes.org.uk
Monday to Friday 9am to 5pm

4. Diabetes UK Publications provide a wide range of information on all aspects of diabetes. For a copy of the Catalogue and other Diabetes UK products, contact:

Diabetes UK Distribution
PO Box 3030, Swindon, Wiltshire SN3 4WN
Telephone: 0800 585 088

Other useful publications

1. About diabetes:
   - *Living with Diabetes*, by Jenny Bryan, published by Hodded Wayland.
   - *Late Onset Diabetes*, by Rowan Hillson, published by Vermilion.
   - *Diabetes at Your Fingertips*, by Sonksen, Fox and Judd, published by Class Publishing.
   - *Diabetes: The Complete Guide*, by Hillsdon, published by Vermilion, London.
2. About nutrition:
   - *Quick and Easy Cooking for Diabetes*, by Asmina Govindji, published by HarperCollins.
   - *Real Food for Diabetics*, by Molly Perham, published by Foulsham.
   - *Diabetes Diet Book: Type 2*, by Calvin Ezrin, published by Contemporary Books Inc.

Medic-Alert

Medic-Alert Foundation

1 Bridge Wharf, 156 Caledonian Road, London N1 9BR
Telephone: 0207 833 3034
Freephone: 0800 581 420

All people with diabetes taking insulin should join Medic-Alert. It is a charity from which identity jewellery, showing that the wearer has a medical condition, may be purchased. A central file on each member is kept at headquarters and the member's doctor may obtain urgent medical information in an emergency. This information can be obtained on making a reverse charge telephone call from anywhere in the world. The telephone is staffed day and night.

Index

acarbose 68
acromegaly 6
activity diaries 93
adherence to lifestyle change,
    promoting 96–7
albumin 21
albuminuria 21
alcohol 13, 76, 103
alopecia 23
anger 36, 38–9
  causes 39
  definition 38
  depression and 36
  exercise and 41
  helpful tips 40–1
  types 38–9
  'why me?' 39
angina 25
annual review 111
antidepressants 38
anxiety 33–4
arthritis 72
atherosclerosis 18, 25–6
attention span 45
autonomic nerves 22
autonomic neuropathy 22

balance of good health
    72, 73
Banting, Frederick 1
Best, Charles 1
biguanides 68
bio-feedback 47
biscuits 74
blood glucose levels 2–3
  in avoidance of hypoglycaemia
    15–16
  measurement of 7

  monitoring 84–5
  personal threshold 85
blood pressure, heart in 25
blood tests 7–8, 84, 85
  nocturnal hypos and 15
blood-testing strips 84
blurring of vision 19

cakes 74
cancer 72
carbohydrate 77
  in alcohol 103
cardiovascular disease 18, 24–5
cataracts 19
causal attribution 31
causes of diabetes 1–2, 5
child teamwork 64–5
children
  effect on 56
  with diabetes 63–5
chiropodists (podiatrists) 24, 109
chocolate 74
coconut oil 74
cognitive behaviour therapy (CBT)
    interventions 94
cognitive distortion 36–7
comments from others, coping with
    61–2
communication 58–9
complications 11
  fear of 49, 50
  long-term 18–26
  short-term 12–18
consultant physician 108
control 31–2
coping
  with child with diabetes 63–5
  with comments from others 61–2

coping (*continued*)
  with depression   35
  fear of failure   51–2
  strategies   32
  with stress   46
corns   24
counselling   51
Coxsackie virus   5
crying   41
Cushing's syndrome   6
cystic fibrosis   5
cystitis   3

dairy foods   73
dancing   77
deep breathing   47, 95
denial   32–3
dependence, fear of   50
depression   34–5
  biochemical causes   38
  coping   35
  exercise and   36
  handling   36–8
  incidence   35
  symptoms   35
diabetes care team   108–9,
    110–11
diabetes clinics   57, 107–8
diabetes specialist nurse   108
Diabetes UK   102, 109–11, 113–14
  Careline   101, 113–14
diabetic foods   76
diabetic ketoacidosis (DKA)   11, 12,
    16
  definition   17–18
  indications   17
  symptoms   18
  treatment   18
diabetologists   108
diagnosis   6–8, 30
diaries, food and activity   93

diet   5–6, 55, 72–3
  aims   72–4
  making changes to   74–6
  need for healthy   71–2
dietitians   109
Disability Discrimination Act (1991)
    (DDA)   101
driving   102–3
Driving and Vehicle Licensing Agency
    (DVLA)   102
driving licence   102

eating out   76–7
emotional reaction to diabetes
    29–30, 32
employment   51, 100–1
endorphins   36
environmental factors   5–6
epileptic fit   14
exercise   78–83
  amount   79, 80, 81
  anger and   41
  as barrier to lifestyle change   96
  depression and   36
  difficulties in   82–3
  effect on insulin   78, 79
  embarrassment   81
  heart and   80–1
  importance in diabetes   79
  need for   79–80
  reasons for   80–1
  stress and   46, 48
eyes   18, 19–20

family   55–6
  indifferent   65
  living with diabetes sufferer
    62–3
  over-indulgent   65
  over-protective   65
fasting plasma glucose test (FPG)
    7–8

fats, dietary
   intake   73–4
   reducing intake   75
   saturated   73–4
   unsaturated   74
fears   49–52
   of injections   49, 59
   of pain   50
   of retinopathy   49
feet   23–4
   blood supply   23
   dryness   24
   expert care   24
   neuropathy   23–4
   shape   24
fight or flight response   44
financial effects   51
fish   73
food diaries   93
friends   50–1, 55, 56
fruit and vegetables   72–3

gastro-enteritis   101
general practitioner   109
gestational diabetes   8
ghee   74
glucagons   12, 14, 15
glucose, blood *see* blood glucose levels
glucose challenge test   8
goals
   setting   59–60
   of treatment   83
guilt   42–3

haemoglobin, glycated   86
HbA1c   86
health-care professionals, relationships
   with   56–60
   consultation   57–8
   negotiating goals   59–60
   partnership   57
   satisfaction with treatment   58–9

heart   24–6
   cardiovascular disease   18, 24–5
   disease   72
   exercise and   80–1
heredity   5
hobbies   48–9
holidays   77
hospital monitoring   85–6
hyperglycaemia   11, 12
   causes   16–17
   definition   16
   symptoms   17
   treatment   17
hypertension   25
hypnosis   31, 47
hypoglycaemia ('hypo')   4, 11,
   12–16
   blood glucose levels and   15–16
   cause   13
   definition   12
   night-time   14–15
   prevention   13
   prolonged   16
   severe   14
   symptoms   12–13
   treatment   14
hypoglycaemic awareness   15
Hypostop   14

illnesses   101
imagery   47
indignation   39
infection as cause of diabetes   5
injection pens   70
injections
   fear of   49, 59
   marks and bruises   70–1
   method   70
   multiple   69
   need for   68
   pain   70–1

insulin   68–71
   discovery   1
   exercise and   78, 79
   hypos and   12, 13
   mechanism of action   3
   resistance   2
   role in hypoglycaemic awareness
      15
   shape   3
   types   69
insurance, motor   102–3
islets of Langerhans   1

ketoacidotic coma   4
ketones   4, 17
kidneys   21

leisure activities, stress and   48–9
lifestyle change   89–97
   action plan   92
   awareness   90–1
   barriers to   95–6
   maintaining   92–3
   making   92
   motivation for   90–3
   preparation for   92
   relapse   92, 93
   stages in   90–3
   strategies for   93–7
   thinking about   91
living with diabetes sufferer   62–3

margarine   74
meals, regular   75
meat   73
Medic-Alert   114–15
medication see insulin; treatment and
      medication
meditation   31, 47, 95
microalbuminuria   21
milk   73
motor nerves   22

motor neuropathy   22
mumps   5
muscle relaxation   95

National Health Service (NHS)
      109–10
National Service Framework for
      Diabetes   110, 113
Naura, Pacific Islanders of   6
necrobiosis lipoidica   23
negative thoughts   37
nerves   22
neuropathy   22
   fear of   49
   feet and   23–4
non-proliferative retinopathy   19

oral glucose tolerance test (OGTT)   8
oral hypoglycaemic agents (OHAs)
      68

paediatrians   108
pain, fear of   50
palm oil   74
pancreas   2, 15
pancreatitis   6
panic   45
parents see family
parties and special events   77–8
peripheral vascular disease   25
podiatrists (chiropodists)   24, 109
polyunsaturates   74
polyuria   3
potassium   18
practice nurse   109
pregnancy   8
prevalence   4
proliferative retinopathy   19–20

Quitline   104

rage   39
random plasma glucose test   8

relapse prevention   95
relationships   50–1
  with family   55–6
  with friends   50–1, 55, 56
relaxation
  exercise and   80
  techniques   44, 47
relief   34
resentment   39
retinopathy   19–20
  fear of   49
  treatment   20–1

salt   75
school   64
Scottish Diabetes Framework
     110
secondary diabetes   6
self-blame   30–1, 42
self-blood glucose monitoring (SBMG)
     84
self-hypnosis   31
self-monitoring   93–4
sensory nerves   22
sensory neuropathy   22
sexual function   22, 46
shared care   108
shift work   100
skin   22–3
  of feet   24
sleep, stress and   49
SMART acronym   60–1
smoking   11–12, 104
snacks   103
social support   95
sports   99–100
  see also exercise
stages of change model   90
starchy foods   72, 75
stigma   50, 61
stimulus control   94

stress   6, 43–5
  causes   45–6
  coping   46
  effect on diabetes   44–5
  effects of   44
  emotional response to
       45–6
  good or bad   45
  helpful tips   47–9
  management   94–5
  response   43, 47–8
  source of   47
  symptoms   44
stress inoculation   95
stressors   43, 48
sugar intake, reducing
     75
sulphonylureas   68, 78
  hypos and   12, 13
swimming   99
symptoms   6–7
  Type 1 (IDDM)   3–4
  Type 2 (NIDDM)   4

thiazolidinediones   68
thrush   3
travelling   51, 77
treatment and medication
  goals of   83
  role of diabetic sufferer in
       83–6
  tablet   68
  Type   1 67
  Type   2 67–8
  see also insulin
treatment plan   86
Type 1 diabetes
  cause   1–2
  genetics   5
  illnesses in   101
  treatment   67–8

Type 2 diabetes
  cause   1–2
  diet and   5–6
  genetics   5
  illnesses in   101
  incidence   4
  treatment   67–8

urine tests   84–5

vegetable oil   74
vitiligo   23

walking   81, 82
weight   5–6
  exercise and   81–2
wheel of change   90
work (employment)   51,
  100–1

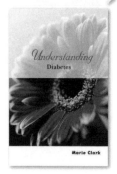
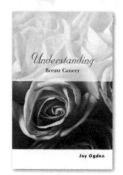
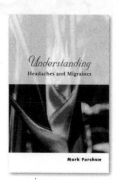